<u>Discovered:</u>
Nature's Secret
Fountains of Youth

A Report from

The American Commission on Anti-Aging

A Hanford Press Research Group

Chief Researcher/Writer:

Robert Concoby, Certified Nutritional Consultant

Editor/Writer: David Nicol

Discovered: Nature's Secret Fountains of Youth
Chief Researcher/Writer:
Robert Concoby, Certified Nutritional Consultant
Editor/Writer: David Nicol

Cover Photo by: Mike Dobel/Masterfile

IMPORTANT:

Table of Contents

Introduction

Chapter 1: The Agents of Aging

Chapter 2: The Anti-Aging Diet

Chapter 3: The Anti-Aging Exercise Plan

Chapter 4: Anti-Aging Skin Care

Chapter 5: Superfoods and Enzymes

Chapter 6: Antioxidants and Anti-Aging

Chapter 7: Minerals and Anti-Aging

Chapter 8: Coenzyme Q10 and Anti-Aging

Chapter 9: Swedish Pollen Extract

Appendix A
UCLA Study Credits Vitamin C with 6 Year Life Extension

Appendix B
Seven Key Energies of Life and Longevity

Appendix C
Antioxidant Enzymes

Appendix D
Swedish Pollen Extract Research

Appendix E
Swedish Flower Pollen Used to Treat Prostatitis

Appendix F
The Cellular Aging Process and Free Radicals

Appendix G
Your Cancer Prevention Plan

Appendix H
Anti-Aging Institutions and Researchers

Bibliography

Introduction

Buried deep within scientific research are many gems of vibrant healthful living. At the American Commission on Anti-Aging, we continually search the entire world for the very best in anti-aging and nutrition research. Using our worldwide network of contacts, we stay on the cutting edge of new technology. As a result, we learn of new information and new health products almost immediately.

To that end, we've read hundreds of research papers, articles, studies, and books to uncover this exclusive information. *Discovered: Nature's Secret Fountains of Youth* represents the completion of Phase 1 of our ongoing research, and is the result of years of study. And yet we've barely scratched the surface.

Unfortunately, most of this vital information remains hidden from the general public. This is largely due to modern medicine's unawareness of these secrets because they choose to follow the medical curative treatment model instead of the nutritional or natural healing pathway.

Doctors spend years in school and clinical education learning the immense field of medicine. And I am glad that they do — all of us have most likely been helped greatly at one time or another by a well-educated, compassionate physician.

But nutrition is largely ignored in the medical school curriculum. Doctors must teach themselves, adding hundreds of hours to their already overfilled schedules. Most doctors simply do not have the time to pursue another specialty. And it would be fair to say that many people have a strong bias against nutrition and the natural preventive model of nutrition.

Doctors who have joined the nutrition ranks admit this lack of education and systemic prejudice. Dr. Elmer Cranton, in the foreword to Dr. Gary Todd's book, *Nutrition, Health and Disease*, stated that he "was amazed to find a very large body of research and well documented scientific knowledge which had been completely ignored in my curriculum at Harvard Medical School. As I increasingly applied these principles in my practice, health benefits were observed which I had not previously believed possible." And I must note at this point that other countries, most notably those in Scandinavia, western Europe and Asia, are years ahead of the U.S. in making health products and anti-aging techniques commonly available to their people.

Today it is possible to live longer. For some, that means more time to enjoy life; for others, it means pursuing goals that will leave their mark on the world.

Some people have taken this search for a longer life to extreme limits: cryonic freezing, elective organ transplantation, and even genetically engineered tissue regeneration.

Let's face it — those people missed the boat. You don't need to be young, rich, or fanatic to look better, feel better, and live longer — maybe much longer — than you normally would. Affordable anti-aging basics are available for anyone. Technology has taken the very best of the natural world and made it quick, simple and easy for all of us to enjoy. Perhaps now we can learn the wise lessons that nature has been trying to teach us all along.

Healthy living remains a continual and satisfying journey. Join us now on that journey. Every technique or nutrient mentioned in this book has been tried and tested in the crucible of human experience. We personally use these secrets every day in our normal routines. The benefits will serve you well for a lifetime — a long, long lifetime.

Robert Concoby, C.N.C.
Canton, Ohio
January, 1993

Chapter 1

The Agents of Aging

At the time of this research no grand theory about the cause of aging has achieved general acceptance. There are, however, a number of factors which have all been shown to contribute to the deterioration of human appearance and well-being.

Recent scientific discoveries have shown how the ill effects of these agents of aging — interruption of the Life-Energy Cycle through mitochondrial starvation, free radicals, cross-linkage and cellular waste accumulation — can be counteracted, prevented, and in some cases reversed. It is these processes that will be the subject of this chapter. The means of limiting the effects or reversing these processes will be discussed in later chapters.

Other factors, such as the effects of genetics and the possible limiting of life span by a yet-to-be-identified "death" hormone, will certainly be the topic of future study but are beyond the scope of this research.

Most of the known "aging processes" can be slowed, prevented and in some cases reversed.

Interruption of the Life-Energy Cycle

All life is dependent on the radiant energy from the Sun. Chloroplasts are the green solar cells of plant life. They collect the light from the Sun and convert that energy into food through the process of photosynthesis. The food is later

FIGURE 1-1
Mitochondria: The Power-Link in the Life-Energy Cycle

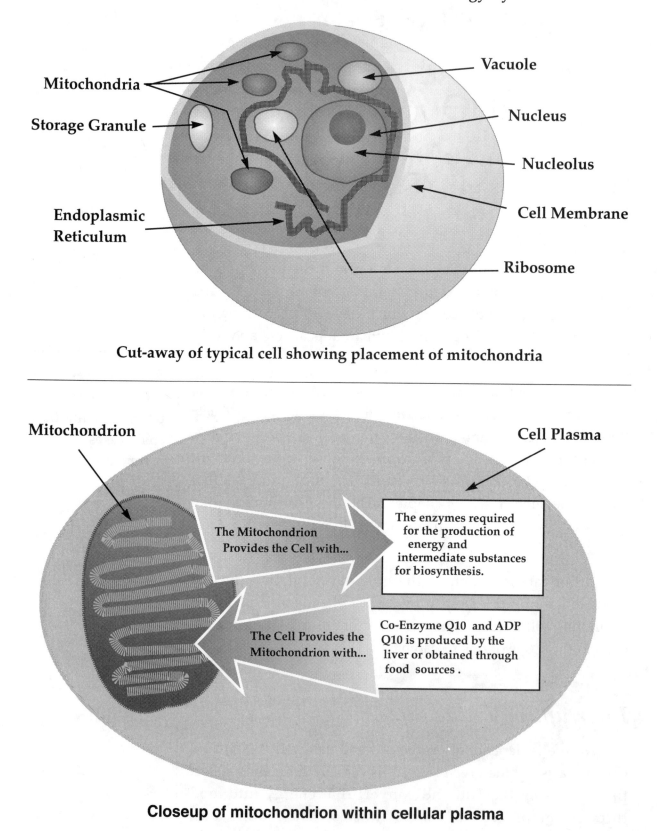

Cut-away of typical cell showing placement of mitochondria

Closeup of mitochondrion within cellular plasma

converted back into energy, by the plant itself, by organisms or animals that eat the plant, or by animals that eat other animals and organisms higher up the food chain.

Part of this Life-Energy Cycle for humans requires bacteria-like structures called mitochondria. Every one of the over ten trillion cells in the body plays host to an average of ten mitochondria. The relationship between these cells and mitochondria is symbiotic, which means that the cell and the mitochondria are beneficially dependent on each other for life.

The host cell provides two essential compounds and a suitable environment for the mitochondria. The mitochondria act as power-plants for the cell — providing the necessary energy for virtually all the cell's processes. One of these compounds is adenosine diphosphate (ADP). As the body

The 100 trillion mitochondria in human cells require Coenzyme Q10 and ADP to do their energy-producing work.

CHART 1-1
Conditions Linked to
Low Mitochondrial Energy Output

- Low levels of Q10. Liver production of this vital enzyme diminishes significantly with age.

- Toxins in system due to bad diet and health endangering habits (drugs, alcohol, tobacco) lower liver's Q10 production.

- Cooking destroys natural enzymes in food.

- Free radical destruction of mitochondrial membranes.

Conditions Associated with Distressed,
Diseased or Starved Mitochondria

Diseases/Disorders	Premature aging symptoms
• Arthritis	• Wrinkles
• Cancer	• Fading Complexion
• Heart Disease	• Age Spots
• Some Degenerative Muscle Diseases	• Loss of Muscle Tone
	• Excessive Weight Gain
	• Low Energy

burns carbohydrates and fats, the mitochondria store all the enzymes required for tricarboxylic acid cycle (TCA) which creates the universal energy molecule, adenosine triphosphate (ATP), from ADP. Then, as the cell needs energy, ATP is

Fountain of Youth Secret No. 1
Coenzyme Q10 is an essential raw material for the body's 100,000,000,000 cellular power plants

converted to ADP, releasing the stored energy. The TCA also produces all the intermdiate substances for bio-synthesis.

To create an energy molecule of ATP, the mitochondria require Coenzyme Q10. This enzyme is normally produced by the liver and supplied to each cell via the blood stream, however, as the liver ages, it produces less and less Q10.

The ATP to ADP conversion produces 95% of the energy required for the processes in the body. At any one time, the body only stores about three ounces of ATP — enough to sustain a strenuous activity for five to eight seconds. That is why Q10 is so important for the maintenance of health and well-being.

Mitochondria that are deficient in Coenzyme Q10 may be the culprit in many so-called "incurable diseases."

An ample supply Q10 keeps the mitochondria replicating and generating the power required by the cell. When mitochondria are deprived of Q10, ATP production slows down and the host cell can no longer derive the energy it needs for vital cellular activities and transactions.

If the situation is not rectified, any or all of the following may occur:

1. The body notices the decrease in energy. Usually the body interprets this loss of energy as hunger. More food is ingested to answer the call, but the nutrients

from the newly ingested food cannot be utilized by the energy-deficient cells. Since the body doesn't use these calories, they are converted to fat and stored.

2. An energy loss weakens the cell and allows it to become prey to microbiological enemies.

3. The cell loses its ability to function properly or ceases to function altogether.

It is believed that this interruption in the Life-Energy Cycle, (enzyme-distressed mitochondria) account for many "incurable diseases."

Damage from Free Radical "Radiation"

Preliminary research suggests that free radicals are a major cause of aging, disease and reduced athletic and mental ability.

Free radicals are fragments of compounds or atoms with missing electrons. They need additional electrons to regain stability and the easiest way to get them is to "steal" them from other atoms and compounds. In the human body, the most available source of electrons is in the large chemically stable molecules in fats, proteins and the genetic materials that make up living tissues.

Unfortunately, as the unstable free radical takes the electrons from a molecule, a new free radical is created. Thus, a chain reaction begins that creates molecular mayhem within the body's intricate systems. Nearly all the damage to the body caused by high-energy radiation — hair loss, skin lesions, skin and organ cancers — is the work of free radicals.

Free radical attack plays a prominent role in the breakdown of plastics, rubber, paper, petroleum and food. Ordinary air on a sunny day contains about one billion hydroxyl free radicals per quart of air. These potent oxidants will attack any organic substance found in cells.

Normal bodily metabolism also creates an abundance of free radicals. Some are normal and necessary. For example, leukocytes (white blood cells) generate free radicals and use

On an ordinary sunny day, an adult will take in over 1,000,000,000 hydroxyl free radicals in every breath.

Nearly all the damage to the body caused by high-energy radiation – hair loss, skin and organ cancers – is the work of free radicals.

them as a major weapon to kill bacteria and viruses. Other free radicals created during bodily metabolism are pathologic and cause damage — such as the breakdown of peroxidized lipids (rancid fats) by radiation.

Carmia Borek, M.D., Columbia University Professor of Pathology and Radiology, states, "Free radical activity may be responsible not just for aging, but for a wide variety of disease states."[1]

According to Joe McCord, Ph.D., a biochemist from the University of Southern Alabama College of Medicine, "The further along we get, the more we are overwhelmed by the number of disease states that involve free radicals. In only a

60 diseases have already been linked to free radical damage including some of the most dreaded.

CHART 1-2

Major Sources of Dangerous Free Radicals

- Radiation – nuclear, electromagnetic, microwaves
- Ozone in air pollution
- Creation of hydroxyls (OH) in air by sunlight
- Metabolism of saturated fats
- Charred and roasted foods – barbequed meat, coffee
- Nitrates and nitrites in processed meats
- Breakdown of hydrogen peroxide in human body
- Herbicides and pesticides
- Rancid fat or food exposed to air during processing such as processed meat, aged cheese, powdered eggs
- Cigarette smoke
- Immoderate consumption of alcohol
- Intense sunlight
- X-rays
- Radon
- Asbestos
- Phenobarbital
- High levels of LDL cholesterol in the blood
- Psychological stress
- Prolonged, exhaustive exercise
- Excess body fat

few cases will free radicals be the whole answer, but they can be important components in many different disorders."[2]

Scientists have now linked 60 diseases with free radicals and are still counting. A great deal of evidence supports the theory that free radical damage is a major factor causing aging, as well as many other disease conditions. Free radicals have been measured in living organisms and it has been shown that they increase in concentration with increasing metabolic rate.

Known changes due to free radicals include:

Free radicals are intimately involved in the conditions associated with aging such as facial wrinkles and stiff joints.

CROSS-LINKING

Free radicals create undesirable bonding and erosion of collagen and elastin. The phenomenon is called cross-linking and is covered in detail in the next subsection. Collagen is the connective tissue which constitutes about 30 percent of body protein) and elastin is an elastic protein found in artery walls and skin. Cross-linking makes tissues stiff and brittle, causing such symptoms as facial wrinkles and sagging jowls. Cross-linking also leads to a loss of flexibility, creating such conditions as emphysema of the lungs and cerebral hemorrhage.

MUTATIONS AND CANCER

DNA and RNA, the genetic blueprints for each cell, can be changed in many undesirable ways by free radicals. These mutations are a major cause of cancer and have been implicated in the genesis of atherosclerotic plaques — a type of tumor.

JOINT LUBRICANT DEGRADATION

Superoxide radicals cause the breakdown of the large carbohydrate molecules that make up joint lubricant. This degradation of joint lubricant is responsible for many of the problems associated with arthritis.

PIGMENT ACCUMULATION

Free radicals cause lipofuscin, proteins and ceroid lipids to accumulate. This accumulation in the skin results in brownish "age spots." In the brain, they slowly choke brain cells to death.

CELLULAR MEMBRANE DAMAGE

Sometimes free radicals attack cellular membranes, with drastic results. Lysosomes, for example, contain powerful enzymes — acid hydrolase — which can dissolve cellular components. When these membranes are ruptured by free radicals, the enzymes are released and cause severe damage to surrounding tissues. Rheumatoid arthritis is an example of this type of attack.

The enzyme xanthine oxidase stimulates the production of both superoxide radicals and hydrogen peroxide, which react together to form hydroxyl radicals. These free radicals, along

Membrane damage to living cells caused by free radicals can render those cell useless. Some of those cells, like neurons and brain cells cannot be replaced.

CHART 1-3

Conditions Linked to Free Radical Damage

- Age Spots from accumulation of pigments.
- Alzheimer's
- Arthritis associated with the degradation of natural joint lubricants.
- Atherosclerotic plaques.
- Brain damage from pigment accumulation.
- Cancer created from DNA and RNA mutation.
- Cerebral hemorrhage due to cross-linking.
- Cross-linking which is responsible for a myriad of other problems (see Chart 1-4)
- Emphysema due to cross-linking.
- Facial wrinkles and sagging jowls due to cross-linking
- Gout
- Heart attack from abnormal blood clotting
- Immune system disruption which lowers resistance to viral infections and bacteria.
- Premature aging due to mitochondrial damage.
- Reduced athletic performance resulting from mitochondrial damage.
- Rheumatoid arthritis
- Stokes from abnormal blood clotting.

---

with crystals of uric acid and sodium hydrogen urate, cause the joint pain and tissue destruction of gout, both directly and by destabilizing the lysosomal membranes.

Fountain of Youth Secret No. 2
Superoxide Dismutase (SOD) — Nature's Anti-Free Radical Mega Weapon

---

Free radicals can also cause red blood cells to burst by breaking their cellular membranes. The measurement of the ease of bursting of red blood cells is a common assay for vitamin E bio-availability, because vitamin E, an antioxidant, can protect the red blood cell membranes.

A damaged membrane can't transport nutrients, oxygen and water into the cell or regulate the removal of waste products. Continued attack renders a cell useless.

ABNORMAL BLOOD CLOTTING

Free radicals can make blood clot abnormally in the arteries by destroying the body's ability to make PGI2 (prostacyclin), a natural anti-clot hormone found in healthy arteries. If there is not enough PGI2, a clot forms on the arterial wall. Iron and copper leak from the bursting red blood cells in the clot and promote the free radical peroxidation of still more fats, further decreasing PGI2, and so the clot grows. After a while, part of the clot may break off. If it lodges in the coronary artery, a heart attack — coronary thrombosis — occurs. If it lodges in the brain, a stroke results and causes brain damage.

DESTRUCTION OF MITOCHONDRIA

Free radical damage to the mitochondria — the cell's power house — limits production of energy and causes

Free radicals can destroy the energy-producing mitochondria and thereby reduce endurance and strength.

accumulation of metabolic fragments or "clinkers." These fragments are associated with reduced athletic performance and premature aging.

Fountain of Youth Secret No. 3
Vitamins A, C and E
SOD and Selenium
Nature's Super Anti-Oxidants

IMMUNE SYSTEM DISRUPTION

Researchers believe that even the immune system, and hence resistance to viral infections and bacteria, may be vulnerable to free radical attack. In fact, unless they are controlled, free radicals have the potential for compromising virtually all the body's life-promoting functions.

THE BODY'S NATURAL FREE RADICAL DEFENSE SYSTEM

The body also has a strong anti-free radical system that, if maintained effectively through diet, can fight off the damage. Two of its weapons, the enzymes superoxide dismutase (SOD) and glutathione peroxidase are substances created by the human liver to control free radicals made in the body. All air-breathing life must have such enzymes to survive.

Superoxide Dismutase — SOD — has been credited with radiodurans' (a bacterium that thrives in nuclear reactors) ability to survive in a lethal environment.

Mammals can produce additional SOD as a response to the presence of increased superoxide radicals. Studies have shown that people living in cities with severe amounts of air pollution, such as LA, Detroit and Denver, have increased amounts of SOD and other protective antioxidant enzymes produced in their bodies. These same people have cancer rates on par with the inhabitants of large cities with relatively clean air.

Dr. Richard Cutler, a noted gerontologist, has performed studies that show the life spans of many mammalian species,

FIGURE 1-2
The Chain-Reactive Nature of Free-Radical Attack

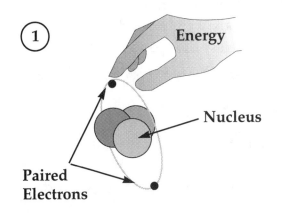

① Energy

Nucleus

Paired Electrons

Energy (light, heat or radiation) or a chemical reaction (oxidation) steals an electron from a stable molecule. Forming a free radical.

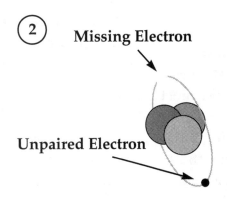

② Missing Electron

Unpaired Electron

Newly created free radical is **unstable because it is missing an electron from its outer shell.**

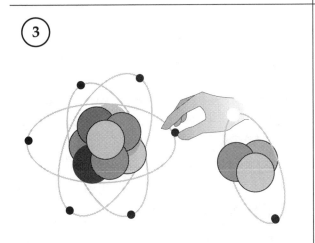

③ The free radical seeks stability by "stealing" an electron, usually from a molecule larger than itself.

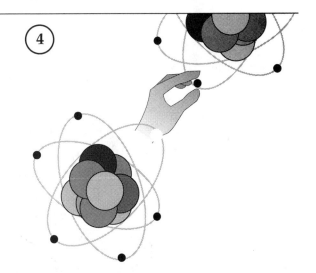

④ This process can continue until **the large molecules in membranes, DNA or RNA are damaged or destroyed.**

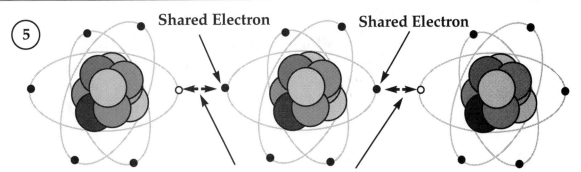

⑤ Shared Electron   Shared Electron

Abnormal Cross-Linking Bonds

Sometimes the large molecules of collagen which have been attracted by free radicals are forced into abnormal bonding in order to satisfy the need for electrons.

including man, are directly proportional to the amount of SOD they contain. These studies also show that life span is inversely proportional to their specific metabolic rate — the number of calories burned per pound of body weight per day. (See Figure 1-2). The animals with the longest life spans have the highest levels of SOD when it is expressed as a function of this metabolic rate.[3]

Further evidence of SOD's ability to limit free radical damage is found in a bacterium called radiodurans. This organism has the highest levels of the enzymes SOD, peroxidase, and catalase ever measured, enabling it to thrive inside nuclear reactors.

Vitamins C, E and the mineral selenium have been shown, in experimental animals, to prevent the development of some types of cancer.

Damage from Cross-Linking

Cross-linking is the progressive formation of chemical links— usually di-sulfide bonds— as bridges between large molecules. As these molecules bond, whether they are in leather, food, plastic, skin, or arterial tissue, there is a loss of flexibility and increase in the tendency to tear. Wrinkled skin is one of the visible manifestations of this process.

When the tissue in arteries becomes cross-linked, they become hard, inflexible, and can no longer pulse normally as the blood is pumped by the heart. Such arteries can cause high blood pressure and are subject to rupture, resulting in internal hemorrhage.

Some cross-linking is necessary to provide structure to certain tissues and organs in the body. Beyond those necessary bridges, additional cross-linking builds up over time and causes damage to organs and tissues, and can even cause life-threatening conditions and diseases.

As a person grows older, one of the most obvious evidences for cross-linking is found in the body's connective tissues. That linkage occurs in the large collagen molecules that makeup approximately 30 percent of the body's protein weight.

As these bonds begin to form, the body loses its elasticity and becomes stiffer. Adults often marvel at the flexibility of babies as they realize their own lack of agility. That process begins shortly after birth and continues until death, bringing about more and more rigidity as the time passes by.

Unfortunately, cross-linking is not limited to connective tissues and skin. It also affects the large protein molecules of DNA and RNA which can restrict a cell's ability to replicate or cause errors in the translation of genetic instructions to the cell, creating an abnormal cell and even resulting in cancer. It is believed that this damage to DNA is a principal cause of aging.

Cross-linking has been tied to cancer and hardening of the arteries.

CHART 1-4
Factors Associated with Cross-Linking

- Free radicals
- Aldehydes — created by smog, cigarette smoking, alcohol consumption
- Ozone
- Ultraviolet light
- X-rays
- Metal ions — from copper, cadmium, aluminum, titanium, lead and a few others.
- Ketones — found in the blood of diabetics.

CHART 1-5
Nutrients That Help Retard Undesirable Cross-Linking

- Anti-oxidants — to mitigate the effect of free radicals.
- Vitamins A, B-1, B-5, B-6, C and E
- Cysteine — an amino acid
- Selenium — a mineral
- Bromelain and papain — protein-digesting enzymes found in raw pineapple and papaya.
- Superoxide Dismutase (SOD)

FIGURE 1-3
The Effects of Cross-Linking

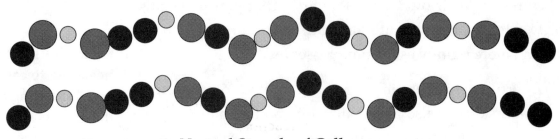

Normal Strands of Collagen
Normal strands in skin, ligaments and tendons are able to stretch and move freely.

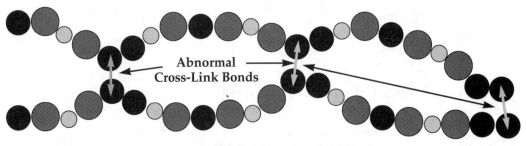

Cross-Linked Strands of Collagen

Abnornal cross-linkage causes a loss of free movement and undesirable structures resulting in stiff joints, loss of flexibility, stretch marks and facial wrinkles — all conditions associated with old age.

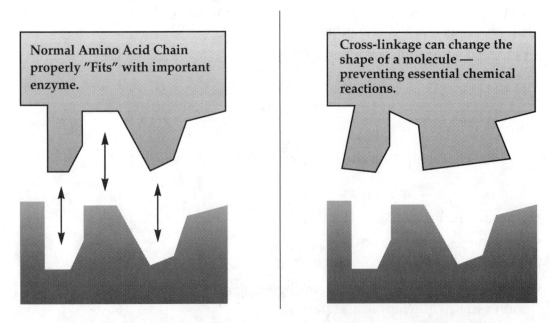

Normal Amino Acid Chain properly "Fits" with important enzyme.

Cross-linkage can change the shape of a molecule — preventing essential chemical reactions.

Abnornal cross-linkage causes a loss of free movement (in joints, ligaments etc.), stretch marks and facial wrinkles.

Several metal ions have been shown to increase cross-linking including cadmium, aluminum, copper and titanium. Heavy metals like lead also promote cross-linking.

Ketones and aldehydes are extremely active in the cross-linking process. Ketones are produced to excess by diabetics and aldehydes are produced by the liver and present in smog and cigarette smoke. These organic compounds typically cross-link unsaturated fats through free radical reactions.

Ultraviolet light, radiation and free radicals are extremely potent cross-linkers. In fact, most of the chemical reactions needed to form damaging cross-linkages require free radical intermediates. Skin receives most of its cross-linking damage at the hands of ultraviolet light.

Researchers believe that the cross-linking process can be slowed and that if the slowing is maintained over a period of several years, a significant amount of the damage can be undone as the body regenerates new tissue. This process takes a long time because structural tissues like collagen are replaced over a period of about seven years or more.

Accumulation of Metabolic Wastes

It has been proposed by some scientists that some parts of the aging process can be explained by the accumulation of metabolic toxic waste products in the body's cells. One of the most visible evidences of this accumulation are called "liver spots" or "age spots." The yellow-brown pigment that comprises these spots is called lipofuscin — a waste material that consists of cross-linked peroxidized lipids and proteins.

Lipofuscin and two other pigments — ceroid and amyloid— accumulate, not only in the skin tissues, but also in neurons, skeletal and heart muscles, the liver, adrenal glands and other organs and tissues that contain fatty compounds. It is believed that aging pigments form in the following manner:

1. Structural components of the cell, especially membranes, are peroxidized by free radical attack.

> **Researchers believe that a significant amount of the damage done by cross-linking can be undone as the body regenerates new tissue.**

FIGURE 1-4
The Damaging Effect of Metabolic Waste Accummulation

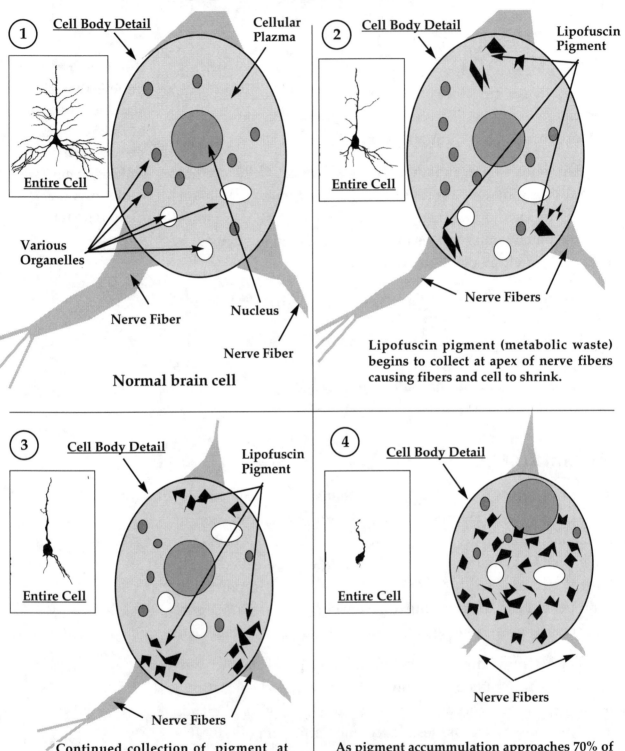

1 <u>Cell Body Detail</u> — Cellular Plazma

<u>Entire Cell</u>

Various Organelles

Nerve Fiber

Nucleus

Nerve Fiber

Normal brain cell

2 <u>Cell Body Detail</u> — Lipofuscin Pigment

<u>Entire Cell</u>

Nerve Fibers

Lipofuscin pigment (metabolic waste) begins to collect at apex of nerve fibers causing fibers and cell to shrink.

3 <u>Cell Body Detail</u> — Lipofuscin Pigment

<u>Entire Cell</u>

Nerve Fibers

Continued collection of pigment at apex of nerve fibers causes more shrinkage of fibers and cell and loss of cell performance.

4 <u>Cell Body Detail</u>

<u>Entire Cell</u>

Nerve Fibers

As pigment accummulation approaches 70% of the cellular volume, the cell will die.

2. The lysosomes, the garbage processors of the cell, engulf these damaged parts and begin to digest them with powerful enzymes. Yet, as strong as the lysosomal enzymes are, they are unable to digest some of all of the damaged tissue.

3. The undigested fragments become the yellow-brown material called lipofuscin and ceroid.

At some point, it is theorized, the cell becomes so cluttered with this debris that it begins to inhibit normal function. Finally, the cell is so filled with this cellular waste that it ceases to function at all. It has been shown that lipofuscin may fill up to 70 percent of cellular volume before the cell perishes.

It has been shown that lipofuscin may fill up to 70 percent of cellular volume before the cell perishes.

Ceroid seems to impair vitamin E absorption and utilization in the liver. Ceroid fragments accumulate quickly in laboratory animals and can become visible in just a few days.

Amyloid is found in the nervous tissues of older humans and patients with various nervous disorders and diseases. The accumulation of amyloid compresses nervous tissues and probably restricts the movement, diffusion movement and reactions of vital biochemicals within the cell.

Much research needs to be completed to fully understand how pigment accumulation contributes to the aging process. It has been shown, however, that aging pigments can be prevented or slowed with the use of antioxidants and/or prescription drugs.

Deterioration of the Immune System

The immune system protects the body from the trillions of deadly micro-organisms that are ever present in the environment. This system is composed of the lymphatic nodes and ducts, the spleen, the bone marrow and the thymus gland. These all work together to produce antibodies, white blood cells and interferon, the body's weapons against these tiny invaders.

FIGURE 1-5
The Human Immune System

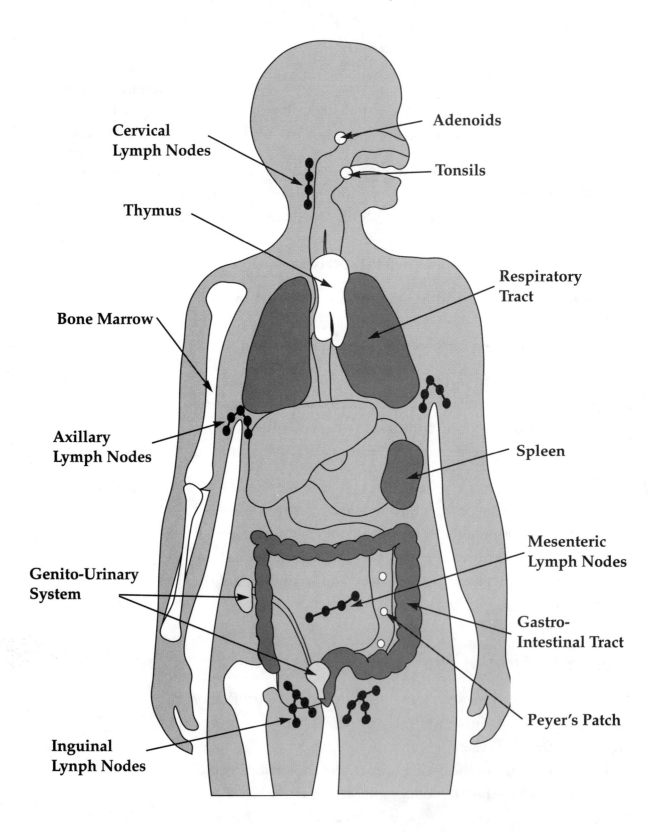

Cervical Lymph Nodes

Adenoids

Tonsils

Thymus

Respiratory Tract

Bone Marrow

Axillary Lymph Nodes

Spleen

Mesenteric Lymph Nodes

Genito-Urinary System

Gastro-Intestinal Tract

Peyer's Patch

Inguinal Lynph Nodes

The thymus gland is a very important part of the immune system. It produces certain white cells — called T-cells — and programs them so they know what to attack and when. Some of the T-cells control the white cells that make antibodies. When the thymus fails to do its work properly, T-cells may fail to attack invading bacteria, viruses and cancer cells. These untrained T-cells have even been known to attack healthy parts of the body, creating auto-immune diseases such as arthritis.

From the point of birth through puberty, the thymus functions at a high level of activity. Shortly after puberty, the thymus slows its production and even begins to shrink. As time passes, the body becomes progressively less able to fight all types of diseases. The diseases associated with age, like atherosclerosis and arthritis, would all be prevented by a well-functioning immune system.

The degeneration of the body's immune system is tied, in large part, to the decrease in growth hormone production by the pituitary gland. At about age fifteen, the pituitary starts to slow its production of growth hormone. Since the thymus requires growth hormone in order to function properly, the reduction in pituitary output produces a serious blow to the immune system.

Growth hormone is normally released — even in adults — in response to sleep, exercise and fasting. Certain nutrients have also been shown to aid the immune system by stimulating the release of growth hormone or by stimulating the thymus gland directly. Some of those nutrients are listed here:

1) **Vitamin E acetate**. In a study conducted by Dr. Cheryl F. Nockels at the University of Colorado, farm and laboratory animals were given mega doses of vitamin E. They reported a tenfold increase in the activity of B-cells, leucocytes produced by the bone marrow, and a three to fivefold improvement in T-cell activity in response to bacteria, viruses and cancer cells.

2) **Vitamin A**. Shown to stimulate the immune system and offer protection to animals from

The diseases associated with age, like arthritis, atherosclerosis and arthritis, would all be prevented by a well-functioning immune system

developing tumors in the presence of some
cancer-causing chemicals.

3) **Arginine and ornithine**. These amino acids,
were able to block formation of tumors in mice
when exposed to a cancer-causing virus. When
these amino acids were added to their food,
there was a significant increase in the mices'
thymus weights and in the production of
lymphocytes and markedly extended survival
time in the mice receiving the cancer virus
inoculation.

4) **Zinc**. Deficiency of this mineral can cause severe
thymus shrinkage, which can be reversed when
zinc is added to the diet. Animal studies
suggest that many humans are probably not
getting enough zinc.

5) **Cysteine and Thiamine (B_1)**. These thiol
compounds, along with others, have been
shown to be effective in stimulating the immune
system. There are other thiol compounds which
are extremely effective but they can cause
damage to the liver if not administered correctly.

6) **Selenium**. This important trace mineral has been
found to act as an anti-carcinogen and anti-
mutagen in experimental animals. Selenium is
also an essential part of the enzyme glutathione
peroxidase, which is important in damage
prevention from free radical oxidation of body
fats and oils.

7) **Vitamin C**. This vitamin increases the activity of
certain white blood cells. It also increases the
quantity of interferon — a substance known to
fight disease. Ten grams per day of vitamin C
has be reported to extend life spans of terminal
cancer patients who had not undergone
immune-suppressing chemotherapy by an
average of over four times.

A Detrimental Lifestyle

Much of the human body's exposure to the agents of aging are a result of a detrimental lifestyle. People choose to smoke, to drink coffee, to live the fast-paced, stress-filled life. They elect to eat too much fat and to consume processed (junk) food by the tons. They also choose not to exercise, not to eat fresh fruits and vegetables, and not to take care of their skin.

Scientists estimate that 68 percent of all cancer deaths are caused by things people do to themselves and each other. Bad diet is blamed for 35 percent of all cancer deaths, smoking for another 30 percent, pollution — air, food and water — for 2 percent and food additives for 1 percent. These preventable cancers involve the bladder, breast, colon, esophageal, larynx, liver, lung, mouth, skin, stomach and uterus.

The objective of this report is to provide the reader with good information so that good choices can be made — choices that will dramatically increase the odds of living a long, energy-filled life free from sickness and disease.

Subsequent chapters will address some of these lifestyle choices and how they affect health and aging. In most cases, minor adjustments can be made which will counteract the ill effects of lifestyle and exposure to harmful environmental factors.

Footnotes

1. Porter Shimer, "Fountain of Youth", *Organic Gardening* (Pennsylvania, Rodale Press)

2. Shimer, *Organic Gardening*

3. Durk Pearson and Sandy Shaw, *Life Extension* (New York, Warner Books), 1982

Chapter 2

The Anti-Aging Diet

Once the factors contributing to premature aging and disease have been isolated and examined (Chapter 1) it becomes very clear that diet has a very important role in the aging process. Eating exposes the body to the largest array of harmful free radicals — one of the chief causes of aging and degenerative diseases. It is also the means for bringing powerful antioxidant nutrients into the body.

Food provides the essential enzymes, amino acids and other nutrients the body needs to repair and replace aging cells. In large part, much of the toxic waste created by metabolism is eliminated through the digestive system with the aid of fiber obtained from food.

Research is now confirming that proper eating and nutrient supplementation can have a dramatic effect on preventing and reversing premature aging — in much the same way poor diet contributes to aging and disease. Unfortunately, the typical American diet is anything but healthful. This fact, in great part, could explain why Americans are the most disease-ridden people in the world.

The data suggests that most Americans cause undue nutritional stress to their bodies because they eat at the wrong times, eat the wrong way, and eat the wrong foods. This chapter will explore these issues and make specific recommendations for improving the diet for optimum life extension.

Americans cause nutritional stress to their bodies because they eat at the wrong times, eat the wrong way, and eat the wrong foods.

When to Eat

For nearly a century, nutritionists and cereal manufacturers have been insisting that Americans eat a large morning meal filled with proteins and complex carbohydrates. Mounting physiological evidence suggests that these traditional concepts about breakfast may be wrong.

Fountain of Youth Secret No. 4
Eating in conformity with the body's circadian rhythm offers many health benefits and could prolong life.

The human body is maintained by a self contained biological clock — sometimes called the circadian rhythm. It is now clear that the major physiological functions take place in defined cycles. For example, the human organism is set up for nocturnal sleep and its physiology is established to function that way. Studies now show that people who work at night and sleep during the day are subject to a large number of physical and emotional disorders.

One of the body's circadian rhythms includes a 24-hour nourishment-elimination cycle.

Research has also shown that there is a definite nourishment/elimination cycle. During every 24-hour period, the body has three distinct and different processes with regard to feeding. Each process follows the next in a logical order and lasts about eight hours. In the same way that an individual can function outside the optimal waking-sleeping cycle, one can also function outside the optimal feeding cycle.

That optimal cycle looks something like this:

Nutrient Ingestion-Digestion:........... **Noon to 8 p.m.**

Nutrient Distribution-Utilization: ... **8 p.m. to 4 a.m.**

Waste Elimination: .... **4 a.m. to noon**

Of the three processes, digestion is the most energy-and resource-demanding. When food is eaten during the optimum ingestion time, the energy and metabolic resources required for digestion are most readily available and their use least interferes with the other two stages of the cycle. When food is eaten outside of this time, energy and materials are taken from the resources needed for one of the other processes, thus hindering efficient completion of either.

It stands to reason that a dietary schedule that works in harmony with the circadian rhythm would promote better digestion, more efficient utilization of nutrients and more complete elimination of waste products. All of these benefits could do nothing but help in the battle against aging.

What to Eat

Scientists are learning more every minute about the physiology of the human body and what it needs to perform properly. Much is already known about the vitamins, minerals, amino acids, enzymes and coenzymes that the body must obtain from outside sources in order to function. As the typical diet is analyzed, it soon becomes apparent that it is woefully lacking in many of these nutrients.

Harvesting foods before they are ripe, freezing, cooking, pasteurizing and other means of processing have been shown to destroy much of the original value of the food before it gets to the table.

This section will provide some suggestions for getting the most out of foods and the best foods to eat to obtain the most anti-aging benefits.

EAT WHOLE, LIVING FOODS

Whole foods are simply foods which still contain all the nutrients nature has put into them — not less and not more. Food processing includes removal or alteration of nutrients or the addition of artificial flavors, colors, emulsifiers, preservatives, etc.. It is estimated that up to 90 percent of the food sold in America has been altered in this way.

Early harvesting, freezing, cooking, and other means of processing have been shown to destroy much of the original value of food before it gets to the table.

FIGURE 2-1
Optimum Food-Group Balance

COMPOSITION OF A HEALTHY DIET

The chart at right represents the optimum breakdown of food intake shown as a percentage of daily caloric intake. This ratio is far different than the typical American diet (see below). Ideally, the vast majority of calories will come from whole, unprocessed foods such as fresh, uncooked fruits and vegetables and whole grains.

The chart in the lower right hand corner shows the optimum composition as a percentage of daily intake by mass (weight).

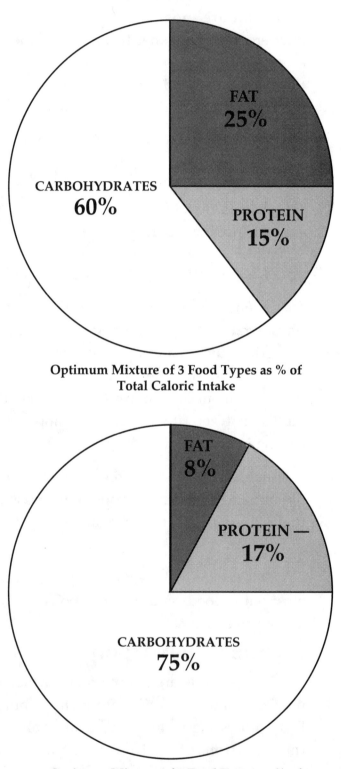

Optimum Mixture of 3 Food Types as % of Total Caloric Intake

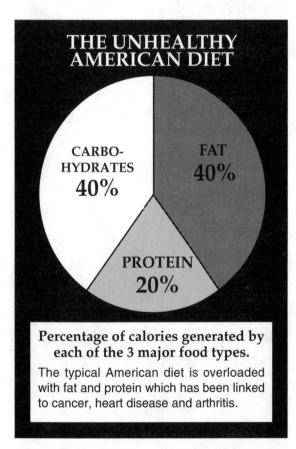

Optimum Mixture of 3 Food Types as % of Total Mass Intake

Processing changes the natural balance of any food. As that balance is disturbed, the food begins to lose its nutritional value. These altered foods have been linked to nutritional deficiencies and health problems in humans, and have been shown, in some cases, to cause premature aging and even death

---

CHART 2-1
Substitution Recommendation for Improving Diet

FAT SUBSTITUTIONS:

Replace...	*...with*
Hard cheeses: like Cheddar, Jack, American, Swiss, Etc.	Soft Cheeses: like Skim Mozzarella, Ricotta, Feta Cheese, Cottage Cheese.
Whole Milk	2% or Skim Milk
Ice Cream	Low or No Fat Frozen Yogurt
Beef, Pork and Processed Meats	Chicken or Turkey without skin or visible fat, fish
Egg yolks	Egg Whites or Egg Substitutes
Solid Cooking Fats like shortening, lard, or bacon fat	Corn oil , safflower oil, soybean oil
Regular Salad Dressing & Spreads	Low Fat or Fat Free Dressing & Spreads
Doughnuts & Pastries	Bagels, English Muffins and Fruits
Chips and Dips	Sunflower Seeds, Whole Wheat Crackers

CARBOHYDRATE SUBSTITUTIONS

Replace...	*...with*
White Sugar	Fructose, Honey
White Flour	Whole Wheat Flour
Soft Drinks	Freshly-Squeezed Fruit Juice
Candy	Nuts and Dried Fruits

in laboratory animals. For example, the use of refined (white) sugar and enriched (white) flour have been tied to the sharp increase in the incidence of diabetes, dental caries, heart disease, ulcers and some cancers.

<u>Fountain of Youth</u> Secret No. 5
Raw and unprocessed foods are chock full of anti-aging nutrients. Eat them and enjoy a long and healthy life.

It is estimated that the human body requires about 600 various enzymes to maintain proper health. Cooking destroys all of them. Cooking also destroys many vitamins and amino acids, also essential to proper nutrition. Prolonged storage, freezing, drying, salting and canning cause a loss to the nutritional value of food.

Japanese and European scientists have demonstrated the powerful anti-aging and disease fighting properties of raw food. Viennese researchers have discovered that raw plant foods increase the micro-electric tension in cell tissue which improves cell metabolism and prevents biochemical suffocation.

An irrefutable amount of evidence is mounting that demonstrates the need to return to unprocessed and uncontaminated foods. Many of the valuable nutrients found in raw food are removed or destroyed by processing and the safety of most additives has not been effectively proven. The pesticides and herbicides used by most industrialized farmers are laden with free radical producing chemicals.

Where possible, fruits, nuts, seeds and vegetables should be eaten raw. Fruits and vegetables should be cleansed thoroughly with mild soap and rinsed with copious amounts of cold water prior to eating to remove harmful chemicals and unwanted micro-organisms.

It is estimated that the human body requires about 600 various enzymes to maintain proper health. Cooking destroys all of them.

CHART 2-2
Best Food Sources for Free-Radical-Fighting Nutrients

Col. A = the quantity of food required to meet the Recommended Daily Allowance (U.S. RDA)

Col. B = the quantity of food recommended by nutritionists for optimum free-radical-fighting benefit.

It is not recommended that a person eat the quantities of food listed but rather this chart is meant to show the value of augmenting normal diet with food supplements.

VITAMIN A

Col. A	Col. B	
1/3 oz.	1 2/3 oz.	Beef Liver
1/3 cup	1 1/3 cups	Dandelion Greens
1/3 cup	1 1/3 cups	Sweet Potatoes
1/3 cup	1 1/3 cups	Dried Apricot
1/3 cup	1 1/3 cups	Pumpkin
1/3 cup	1 1/3 cups	Cooked Spinach
1/2 cup	2 cups	Collards
1/2 tbs.	2 tbs.	Dried Red Peppers
1/2 cup	2 cups	Raw Watercress
1 cup	4 cups	Cooked Kale

VITAMIN C

Col. A	Col. B	
1 1/2 oz.	1/2 cups	Currents
4 oz.	4 cups	Strawberries (frozen)
3 1/2 oz.	3 2/3 cups	Brussel Sprouts
4 oz.	4 cups	Orange Juice (fresh)
4 1/3 oz.	4 1/2 cups	Lemon Juice
4 3/4 oz.	4 2/3 cups	Papaya
5 oz.	5 1/3 cups	Grapefruit Juice
2 lbs.	17 lbs.	Green Peppers
1/3 whole	2 3/4 whole	Cantaloupe
5 1/2 oz.	5 3/4 cups	Collards

VITAMIN E

Col. A	Col. B	
1 1/3 Whole	22 1/4 Whole	Sweet Potato
65 halves	432 halves	Walnuts
46 spears	307 spears	Asparagus
1 cup	6 2/3 cups	Sunflower Seeds
7 whole	467 whole	Almonds
63 whole	417 whole	Hazelnuts
38 whole	250 whole	Brussel Sprouts
12 1/2 cups	83 1/3 cups	Broccoli
2 cups	14 cups	Wheat Germ
17 whole	111 whole	Apple (medium)

CALCIUM

Col. A	Col. B	
4 oz.	4 oz.	Swiss Cheese
3 cups	3 cups	Milk, whole or skim
3 cups	3 cups	Yogurt, low fat
3 1/3 cups	3 1/3 cups	Tofu
4 cups	4 cups	Turnip Greens
1/2 lb.	1/2 lb.	Sardines, in oil
1 lb.	1 lb.	Salmon, canned, pink
6 cups	6 cups	Kale
10 cups	10 cups	Broccoli
10 cups	10 cups	Navy Beans

MAGNESIUM

Col. A	Col. B	
3 lbs.	3 lbs.	Cod Steak
3 1/2 cups	3 1/2 cups	Lima Beans
3 cups	3 cups	Black-eyed Peas
3 cups	3 cups	Garbanzo Beans
12 1/2 cups	12 1/2 cups	Whole Milk
3 1/3 cups	3 1/3 cups	Granola
6 1/4 cups	6 1/4 cups	Oatmeal
3 1/2 whole	3 1/2 whole	Avocado
36 whole	36 whole	Dried Figs
4 cups	4 cups	Broccoli (cooked)

ZINC

Col. A	Col. B	
3/4 lb.	3/4 lb.	Beef Chuck
3 lbs.	3 lbs.	White Meat Chicken
6 steaks	6 steaks	Salmon
1 whole	1 whole	Raw Eastern Oyster
7 cups	7 cups	Split Peas
20 whole	20 whole	Chicken Eggs
6 2/3 cups	6 2/3 cups	Whole Milk
1 1/4 lbs.	1 1/4 lbs.	American Cheese
11 cups	11 cups	Bran Flakes
13 1/2 cups	13 1/2 cups	Brown Rice

Compiled from The COMPLETE BOOK OF VITAMINS & MINERALS a Consumer Guide® Publication and
THE COMPLETE GUIDE TO ANTI-AGING NUTRIENTS by Sheldon Saul Hendler, M.D., Ph.D

Cereals, grains and breads should be eaten in their complete form — any that claim to be fortified or enriched should be avoided. Processed meats and processed and pasteurized dairy products should be eliminated from the diet altogether.

Fountain of Youth Secret No. 6

Reduce animal proteins in the diet and avoid eating proteins and starches together in the same meal.

REDUCE ANIMAL PROTEIN IN DIET

One conclusion about diet that offers some massive anti-aging benefit runs counter to popular American thought. However, startling and conclusive research has shown:

1) Americans eat more animal protein than any other people.

2) Americans are the most disease-ridden people in the world.

3) American Seventh-Day Adventists, who are predominately vegetarians, live an average of seven years longer than their meat-eating peers.

4) All cultures that are known for their good health and longevity eat very little animal protein and an abundance of natural complex carbohydrates.

All cultures that are known for their good health and longevity eat very little animal protein and an abundance of natural complex carbohydrates.

How to Eat

Civilized man is the only creature on earth who sits down to eat a seven course meal of highly processed foods from four major food groups. From a physiological perspective this dietary habit is unnatural and probably unhealthy. Different foods require different enzymes and produce different degrees of acidity or alkalinity as they are digested. They also require a different amount of time in the stomach for thorough digestion. Based on the physiology of digestion, the following dietary regimen is recommended.

FRUITS AND FRUIT JUICES

The natural attributes of fresh fruit make it the ideal food for early morning breakfast and as a mid-afternoon snack.

Because fresh fruit contains many of the enzymes required for human digestion, it requires much less time in the stomach. Even though fruit generally contains weak acids, it also tends to neutralize the strong digestive acids in the stomach. For this reason, it is recommended that fruit be consumed alone — at

The combining of starches and animal proteins in the stomach is unnatural and unhealthy.

Fountain of Youth Secret No. 7
Limit eating to fresh fruits and fresh fruit juices from the time you wake until noon.

---

least 30 minutes before other food and at least 3 hours after other food.

Much of the nutritional value in fruit is in its enzymes. Since enzymes are destroyed by heat, fruit is much more nutritious when it is uncooked. Canned fruit and canned or frozen juices have been cooked, so for optimal benefit, juice should be freshly squeezed.

PROTEINS AND STARCHES

The typical diet is filled with starch and protein combinations — meat and potatoes, cheese and pasta, pancakes and bacon. This combination can be disastrous in the stomach for the following reasons:

1) Proteins, especially those from animal sources, require highly acidic digestion. Anything that would tend to neutralize the strong digestive juices in the stomach, such as fruit, starches, and liquids, will slow digestion. When this happens, a significant amount of undigested meat can pass into the small intestines and begin to decay, causing some serious toxicity problems.

2) Starches require alkaline digestion. When combined with the strong acids required to digest animal proteins, sugars and starches tend to ferment, accounting for much of the sluggish and drowsy feelings that often accompany a large meal of meat and starch.

It is therefore recommended that nuts, seeds, and meats be eaten alone or mixed with low starch vegetables. And, in like manner, high starch vegetables and grains be eaten alone or mixed with vegetables.

Fat and charred food both produce great numbers of free radicals. Visible fat should be removed from red meat and poultry before cooking, and charring meat should be avoided.

VEGETABLES

Leafy vegetables, root-type vegetables and head-type vegetables should be eaten raw. If the palate prefers them cooked, steam or stir fry instead of boiling. Boiling will leach out the water soluble vitamins and organic minerals important for good nutrition.

Vegetables should be freshly picked and cleaned before eating. Wash them thoroughly with mild soap and water to remove residual pesticides and herbicides, then rinse with large amounts of cold water.

Starchy vegetables like dry beans, potatoes, and grains can be mixed with other vegetables but should not be mixed with animal proteins. All grains should be eaten in the whole form — with the bran.

WATER AND BEVERAGES

Distilled water is preferred over tap water for drinking and cooking — regardless of its origin. Tap water contains a host of free radicals and free radical producing chemicals, and the minerals in water are inorganic (not living) and not usable by the body.

Fountain of Youth Secret No. 8

Fast one or two times a week to help eliminate metabolic wastes and extend life.

Although most Americans do not drink enough water, too much liquid in the diet can be almost as detrimental as too little. The amount of water needed varies with temperature and activity. A glass of water upon waking is advisable; afterwards, drink only when thirsty.

Liquids should not be consumed during a meal or within a couple of hours after a meal because the liquid will dilute the stomach secretions and hinder digestion.

FASTING

Much research has been done with laboratory animals that shows moderate over-eating shortens life and moderate under-eating prolongs life. In one study, underfed rats lived almost twice as long as their regularly fed peers.

Fasting also stimulates the production of growth hormone by the pituitary, which is instrumental in stimulating the immune system. The old adage of "starving a fever" is great advice to those suffering with the flu or minor infections.

Although no human studies have been done to substantiate this effect for humans, most nutritionists agree that

Americans are overfed. Fasting has also been shown to be effective in ridding the body of toxic wastes. One of the predominant theories of aging claims that many diseases and signs of aging are the result of metabolic waste accumulation.

It is believed by some that fasting one or two days a week could add several health-filled years to the average American life span. (Note: one should consult a physician before beginning any type of fasting program.)

The Dangers of Cigarette Smoking

Second only to bad diet in causing cancer, cigarette smoking is one of aging's most effective agents. Smoking claims over 6,000 lives each day — 2.5 million per year. It introduces trillions of free radicals into the human lung, liver and blood stream. Cigarette smoke causes cross-linking in the arteries (hardening of the arteries) and on the skin (wrinkles).

Almost nothing a person can do has more damaging effects on the health and life span. Cigarette smoke contains over 3000 different chemicals — most of which are toxic (see chart 2-3). And, secondhand (or side stream) smoke is even more toxic than the smoke inhaled by the smoker.

The following diseases and conditions have been associated with cigarette smoking:

- Alzheimer's
- Bronchitis
- Collapse of Blood Vessels
- Destruction of Taste Buds
- Fetal Death
- High Blood Pressure
- Impotence in Men
- Spontaneous Abortions

- Birth Defects
- Cancer
- Damage to DNA
- Emphysema
- Heart Disease
- High Blood Sugar
- Infertility in Women
- Ulcers

CHART 2-3
Seventeen of the 3,000+ Chemicals Present in Cigarette Smoke

Acrolein — A toxic, colorless liquid with irritating cancerous vapors.

Acetaldehyde — A highly toxic, flammable liquid that irritates the eyes and mucous membranes and accelerates the action of the heart. Prolonged exposure causes blood pressure to rise and causes proliferation of white and red blood cells.

Acetonitrile — A toxic compound found in coal tar and molasses residue and used in the production of plastics, rubber, acrylic fiber, insecticides and perfumes.

Ammonia — A gaseous alkaline compound of nitrogen and hydrogen used as a coolant in refrigerating and air conditioning equipment, and in explosives, artificial fertilizers and disinfectants.

Arsenic — A highly toxic element used in some rat poisons.

Carbon Monoxide — A highly toxic, flammable gas used in the manufacture of numerous chemical products. Inhalation of carbon monoxide interferes with the transportation of oxygen from the lungs to the tissues, where it is required.

Formaldehyde — A pungent gas used primarily as a disinfectant and preservative. It is extremely irritating to the mucous membranes.

Formic Acid — A pungent liquid gas used in processing textiles and leather. Exposure to the acid irritates the mucous membranes and causes blistering.

Hydrogen Cyanide — An extremely poisonous liquid used in many chemical processes including fumigation, and in the case-hardening of iron and steel. Hydrogen cyanide gas is used as the lethal agent in capital punishment.

Hydrogen Sulfide — A poisonous gas produced naturally from putrefying matter and used extensively in chemical laboratories.

Methanol — A poisonous liquid alcohol used in automotive antifreezes, rocket fuels, synthetic dye stuffs, resins, drugs and perfumes.

Methyl Chloride — A toxic gas used in the production of rubber and paint remover and as an antiknock agent in gasoline.

Nicotine — A poisonous alkaloid that is the chief addictive substance in tobacco. It is also used as an insecticide and to kill parasitic worms in animals. One pack of cigarettes a day, inhaled, provides enough nicotine to kill a person outright if it were given in a single dose.

Nitrous Oxide — A group of irritating and sometimes poisonous gases that combine with hydrocarbons to produce smog. Nitrogen dioxide can weaken bodily tissues and increase susceptibility to respiratory ailments.

Phenol — A caustic, poisonous acidic compound present in coal and wood tar and used in disinfectants.

Propionaldehyde — A colorless liquid with a suffocating odor, used as a chemical disinfectant and preservative as well as in plastic and rubber.

Pyridyne — A flammable liquid used in pharmaceuticals, water repellents, bactericides, and herbicides.

Chapter 3

The Anti-Aging Exercise Plan

Studies conducted at the Human Performance Laboratory at the University of California, Los Angeles, have revealed important information about fitness and aging. That information, once applied, can bring life lengthening health to people everywhere.

Cardiovascular fitness, or the lack of it, has a tremendous impact on the body's ability to stay young and healthy. The lungs, the heart, the muscles and the skeleton all benefit from adequate conditioning and they all aid in the transport of nutrients to all parts of the body. They are all involved in elimination of metabolic wastes as well.

Cardiovascular fitness, or the lack of it, has a tremendous impact on the body's ability to stay young and healthy.

According to some recent studies, people who exercise are less likely to get cancer. In three different studies, researchers discovered the following relationships of exercise and cancer:

1) Active people were more cancer-free than moderate exercisers, who were less likely to have had cancer than sedentary types.

2) Former college athletes have a lower lifetime occurrence rate of cancer than their nonathletic peers.

3) Nonathletes had almost double the risk of breast cancer and over double the risk of reproductive system cancer as did former athletes.

Some scientists believe that exercise reduces cancer risks because it reduces obesity, reduces estrogen levels (in women) and that exercisers generally have a healthier lifestyle.

Three other studies have found that men with physically active jobs are less likely to get cancer — carpenters, plumbers,

Fountain of Youth Secret No. 9

A regular exercise program can dramatically reduce the risk of getting cancer.

gardeners, and mail carriers are at less risk than bookkeepers, accountants and lawyers.

Fitness Myths

Many misconceptions have kept people from the kind of diet and exercise that could keep them fit and healthy. Here are a few:

1) No pain, no gain.

2) A person has to sweat to get in shape.

3) Big muscles make a person stronger.

4) Protein makes a person strong.

5) A person must spend at least ten hours a week in a fitness program to get and stay in shape.

Certainly the fitness requirements of a professional boxer differ from those of an accountant in the conditioning that is necessary to maintain efficient job performance. But, the fitness requirements for either to live and function in a normal way, assuming the same age, gender and weight, are nearly identical.

It is this aspect of fitness, maintaining the level of conditioning necessary to allow the proper functioning of all bodily processes, that will be discussed in this chapter.

A Lesson from Space

In the early 1960s, NASA was working toward putting a man on the moon. During that time, a fitness program was developed that would allow astronauts to work in a weightless environment for 28 days, return to Earth and still have the ability to function.

Working in a gravity-free space lab presents a real problem. For without gravity, it is extremely easy to perform normal activities — so easy in fact, it requires almost no effort at all. Within 28 days, without a special fitness program, astronauts would lose eighty percent of their fitness, and would need to be carried from the space capsule on a stretcher upon their return to Earth.

The scientists who were assigned to the space fitness program were faced with the problem of knowing if the prescribed fitness program was strenuous enough to keep the

Eighty percent of an individual's fitness can be gained or lost in a 28 day period.

CHART 3-1

Heart Rate in Relation to Perceived Exertion

<u>Pulse Rate</u>	<u>Scale of Perceive Exertion</u>
Under 90	Very, very light
90	Light
100	Light
110	Fairly light
120	Moderate
130	Somewhat heavy
140	Heavy
150	Very heavy
160	Very, very heavy

---

astronauts conditioned, and yet not so difficult as to over-tax their systems.

It was through this program that the scientists discovered each astronaut had their own internal computer which constantly monitored his individual level of conditioning and fitness. They learned that by simply monitoring the heart beat, the level of effort and fitness could be determined at any point in time.

Later, it was determined that this continual gauge of fitness is effective for all humans, whether in space or on the Earth, whether ten years old or eighty years old, whether male or female.

Pulse Rate — The Fitness Monitor

The pulse is a constant and accurate indicator of cardio-vascular condition and the degree of effort being expended by

---

CHART 3-2
Training Heart Rates — Beats/10 Seconds

	Training Heart Rate		
Age	**1st Stage**	**2nd Stage**	**3rd Stage**
25-35	19	22	25
36-45	18	21	24
46-55	17	20	23
56-65	16	19	21
66-75	15	18	20
76-85	14	17	19
86-95	13	16	18

1st Stage = 0 - 8 weeks of continuous tri-weekly exercise
2nd Stage = 8-16 weeks of continuous tri-weekly exercise
3rd Stage = 16+ weeks of continuous tri-weekly exercise

the body. In general, the lower the resting heart rate, the better the health and conditioning of an individual. In fact, the mortality rate for adults with resting pulse rates over 92 is four times greater than for those with pulse rates less than 67.

Heart rate increases in direct proportion to the amount of exertion being placed on the cardio-vascular system. An accelerated heart beat indicates more bodily stress; a lower rate indicates less bodily stress. As fitness improves, resting pulse

The mortality rate for adults with resting pulse rates over 92 is four times greater than for those with pulse rates less than 67.

CHART 3-3
Activities that will burn 300 calories

Activity	Distance or Time
Basketball	36 minutes
Bicycling	8.6 miles
Bowling (continuous)	45 minutes
Chopping Wood	45 minutes
Dancing (square)	50 minutes
Ditch-digging	45 minutes
Football	36 minutes
Gardening	1-1/3 hour
Golf	1-1/4 hour
Handball	30 minutes
Horseback riding (trot)	50 minutes
Housework	1-2/3 hours
Rowing (machine)	25 minutes
Running	2.5 miles
Skating (ice)	45 minutes
Skating (roller)	50 minutes
Skiing (snow, 10 mph)	30 minutes
Skiing (water)	38 minutes
Stacking heavy objects (logs, boxes)	50 minutes
Swimming	1 hour
Table tennis	52 minutes
Tennis	42 minutes
Typing	2.5 hours
Volleyball	50 minutes
Walking	3.5 miles

rate lowers, the pulse becomes stronger and it requires more strenuous exercise to achieve a pulse over 120.

Achieving and Maintaining Fitness

The key, then, to achieving fitness and thereby prolonging life expectancy, lies in lowering the at-rest pulse rate. That rate,

---

Fountain of Youth Secret No. 10

Fitness can be achieved in as little as 30 minutes per week with this Anti-Aging Fitness Plan

---

in large part, is determined by the level of activity that has been maintained during the last four weeks.

To illustrate this principle, consider an individual who has lived an entirely sedentary life for thirty years. Then, for the next four weeks enroll him in a fitness program like the one outlined in this chapter. At the end of the four-week period, he would be within 20 percent of total cardiovascular fitness. His resting heart rate would be lower, his muscles would have better tone and his calorie-burning metabolism would be stepped up.

A person who hasn't exercised a bit in 20 years can regain total fitness in three 10-minute sessions a week.

This means that most people are closer to cardiovascular fitness than they realize. According to Laurence E. Morehouse, Ph.D., founding director of the Human Performance Laboratory at U.C.L.A., there are five daily requirements for maintaining fitness:

1) Limbering — 2 or 3 minutes of simple stretching, twisting, bending and turning.

2) Standing for a total of 2 hours during the day.

3) Lifting something heavy for at least 3 minutes.

FIGURE 3-1
How to Measure Heart Rate

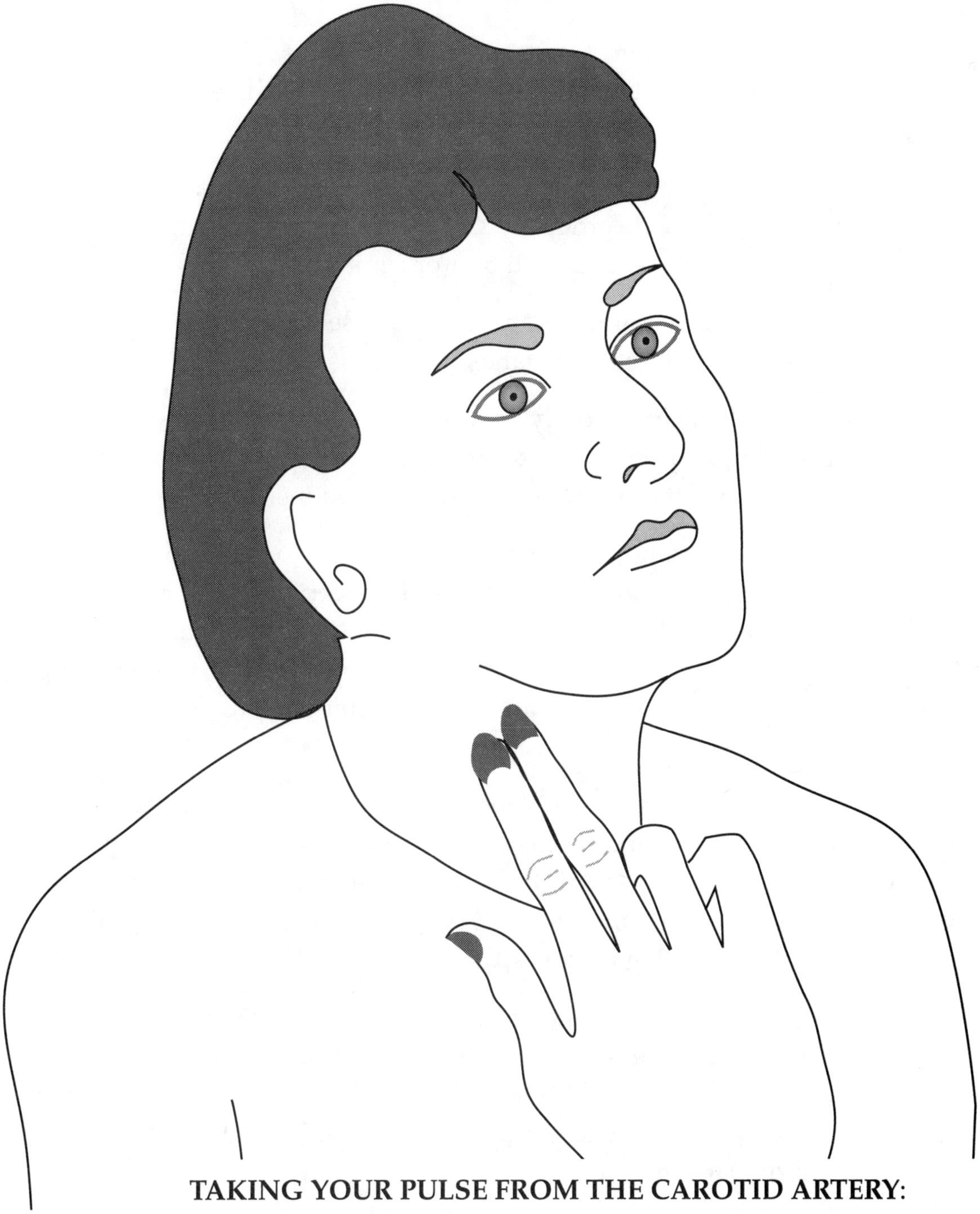

TAKING YOUR PULSE FROM THE CAROTID ARTERY:

1. Place your third and index fingers on the neck, as shown, just behind the larynx and push in.

2. At rest heart-rate should be measured at least 30 minutes after strenuous activity and at least 5 minutes of sitting without talking.

3. Active heart-rate should be always be measured while jogging or walking in place.

4) Walking briskly for at least 3 minutes.

5) Calorie burn — an activity that will utilize at least 300 calories a day.

In addition, two tri-weekly activities which will require approximately 10 minutes on each of 3 different days are necessary:

1) Five minutes of exercise that works the major muscle groups — upper body, abdominals and legs — preceded by 1 or 2 minutes of warm up.

2) Five minutes of aerobic exercise that gets the pulse into the target range (see Chart 3-2).

Exercising every other day is more effective than a daily workout.

Most of the daily requirements can be met — without setting a special time to exercise — simply by incorporating these activities into the normal daily routine.

For example, during a shopping trip to the grocery store, a person will normally twist to look for certain items, bend to get an item of the bottom shelf, stretch to get something of the top shelf — that meets requirement number one. If the shopping trip takes more than an hour, the standing requirement will have been met.

Most fitness requirements can be worked into the normal daily routine.

Carrying in the groceries will take care of the lifting requirement and if it is done briskly, it will meet requirement number four. And, if this is a prolonged trip (two hours or so), all five requirements might be met. (See Chart 3-3 for a list of calorie burning activities.)

Studies have shown that aerobic exercise has more value when done every other day than when done every day. Therefore, the tri-weekly activities should be done on a Monday-Wednesday-Friday, or Tuesday-Thursday-Saturday, or a similar configuration.

The first section of the tri-weekly routine can be accomplished with push-ups, sit-ups and deep knee bends; the second phase by following along with an aerobic dance video as long as the pulse stays around the target range for at least five minutes.

During Stage One — (the first eight weeks), the muscle workout should be done using slow, deliberate movements (approximately ten repetitions of each exercise) and the aerobic portion should get the pulse rate up to but not exceeding the Stage One Target.

During Stage Two — (the second eight weeks), the muscle workout should be done using faster, but deliberate movements (approximately fifteen repetitions of each exercise) and the aerobic portion should get the pulse rate up to but not exceeding the Stage Two Target.

During Stage Three — (the third eight week period and beyond), the muscle workout should be done with the goal of doing as many repetitions as possible within the five minutes. The aerobic portion should get the pulse rate up to but not exceeding the Stage Three Target.

Chapter 4

Anti-Aging Skin Care

The Importance of Skin Care

The skin is the body's largest organ. Aside from protecting the muscles and internal organs from exposure to dangerous environmental factors, the skin plays a critical part in the body's waste elimination processes.

Nearly one third of all bodily wastes are eliminated through the sweat glands of the skin — over one pound of wastes per day. Hundreds of thousands of these sweat glands act like small kidneys, detoxifying organs, ready to cleanse the blood and free the system from health-threatening toxins. The chemical makeup of sweat is very similar to that of urine.

When the skin becomes inactive and its pores clogged with millions of dead cells, uric acid and other impurities will remain in the body.

In addition to its eliminative work, skin has many other vital functions. The body actually breathes through the skin, absorbing oxygen and exhaling carbon dioxide which is formed in the tissues. Scientific studies have also demonstrated that the skin absorbs and assimilates various vitamins, minerals, and even proteins applied directly to the surface.

Skin also manufactures vitamin D when sunlight reacts with the oils produced by skin glands. Subsequently, vitamin D is absorbed into the system through the skin.

When the skin becomes inactive and its pores clogged with millions of dead cells, uric acid and other impurities will remain in the body.

Ultraviolet radiation, which comes predominately from the sun, penetrates the skin and disorganizes the cells.

Failure to give proper care to this valuable organ soon takes its toll on an individual's appearance. As aging progresses, the skin shows the results of aging damage by becoming wrinkled and losing its elasticity. Skin neglect has also been linked to premature aging for the entire body.

The skin is subject to most, if not all, aging factors that attack the internal organs and systems. It has been shown that the appearance of the skin is an accurate representation of what's happening internally.

Nerve cells are derived from the same fetal cells as the skin and these two types of tissue have much in common biochemically. Both skin and nerve cells can accumulate age pigments and become cross-linked. And, both are stimulated to grow by hormones that are very similar. With the exception of ultraviolet light damage from the sun, the skin is a window to what's happening to the neural cells in the central nervous system and the brain.

Only the brain and the spinal cord have more fatty tissue than the skin. As a result, these three areas are particularly susceptible to free radical attack. Studies have shown that people with a greater exposure to cross-linkers, such as alcohol, tobacco, smoke, and sunlight, are more wrinkled. The greater the exposure, the greater the wrinkling. People who smoke and drink heavily usually look old beyond their years.

This chapter will discuss the major factors which cause premature aging of the skin and some of the ways to counteract them.

The Sun — Skin's Worst Enemy

Ultraviolet radiation, which comes predominately from the sun, penetrates the skin and disorganizes the cells. Ultraviolet B (UVB), the shorter rays, burn the skin, and Ultraviolet A (UVA), the longer rays, have been shown to cause aging damage. Both UVA and UVB create free radicals which can damage the cell's DNA and start the formation of cancer.

UV light also causes the lipids in exposed skin to undergo several types of free radical damage, including peroxidation and cross-linking reactions (see chapter one). There is now indirect evidence that UV light attacks the immune system, making the body more susceptible to allergies, disease and aging.

Fountain of Youth Secret No. 11
The skin should be protected from dangerous UV light with a sun screen containing PABA

One way to protect the skin from UV damage, other than staying out of the sun, is found in a vitamin called PABA — p-aminobenzoic acid. PABA and its esters shield the skin by absorbing the energy from UV light. The most effective use of PABA is in the use of topical sun-blocking lotions that contain it. Large oral doses of PABA have been shown to be somewhat effective at preventing sun damage as well.

Oral doses of beta carotene are effective at protecting the the skin from UV light. Beta carotene is converted to vitamin A by the body as needed and is sometimes prescribed by doctors to those who have a particular sensitivity to sunlight. Large amounts of this substance are not toxic but have been known to turn the skin yellow.

Beta carotene is sometimes prescribed by doctors to those who are particularly sensitive to sunlight.

Chlorinated Water and the Skin

Most municipalities add chlorine to public water as a disinfectant. A problem arises when chlorine combines with the natural organic matter in the water — dead leaves and humus in the soil, silt, and mud. This chemical reaction creates a group of volatile pollutants known as trihalomethanes (THMs). The most common THM is chloroform, which can cause liver and kidney damage, central nervous system depression and is a suspected human carcinogen.

According to the Environmental Protection Agency, THMs are present in virtually all chlorinated water supplies in the

Fountain of Youth Secret No. 12

An inexpensive shower filter can protect the skin from damage and toxins created by chlorinated water.

United States. The EPA reports that THMs can liberate themselves from water via mist and steam to become air pollutants. This was discovered while doing a study of indoor pollution. High levels of chloroform were consistently found inside homes and were ultimately traced to hot running shower water.

A 15-minute shower or bath puts nearly twice the volatile contaminants (like THMs) into the body as one would get from drinking two quarts of the same water.

In Chapter Three, the merits of drinking distilled water are discussed, so that issue will not be discussed here. But, researchers say that a normal adult, taking a 15-minute shower or bath each day, is exposed to nearly twice as much of a volatile contaminant (like THMs) in the water as from drinking two quarts of the same water. Researchers say that these figures are based on very conservative estimates and do not take into account a number of factors known to increase skin absorption, such as wetness of the skin, higher temperatures, breaks in the skin and the use of soap.

One way to eliminate the emission of THMs from chlorinated shower water is the use of a simple filter that attaches to the showerhead. Those specifically designed to remove chlorine are filled with KDF, a high purity copper/zinc alloy. Instead of absorbing the chlorine like activated carbon filters, KDF transforms the chlorine into chloride salts.

Diet and the Skin

Most of the nutrients that have been shown to be helpful in retarding the aging process in the body are also helpful in reducing the effects of aging in the skin. Vitamins A, C, E, B1, B5, B6, the mineral selenium, and the amino acid cysteine, have been shown to slow the rate of cross-linking — the cause of wrinkling in the skin. Foods rich in these substances should be included in the daily diet, not only for healthy skin but for healthy bodies (see Chapter Three).

Raw pineapple and raw papaya contain large amounts of protein-digesting enzymes. When these fruits are eaten fresh, significant quantities of these protein dissolvers end up in the blood. Some cross-linked as well as some non-cross-linked proteins will be dissolved by these enzymes. The body will replace the dissolved proteins with non-cross-linked proteins. These fruits are not recommend for people with ulcers.

It has been suggested that applying raw pineapple or papaya directly on wrinkled skin may help to dissolve this

Most of the nutrients that have been shown to be helpful in retarding the aging process in the body are also helpful in reducing the effects of aging in the skin.

Fountain of Youth Secret No. 13

The enzymes found in raw pineapple and papaya can dissolve the cross-linked proteins that cause wrinkles.[1]

---

cross-linked collagen over a period of time. The body will replace the old cross-linked collagen with new, more elastic, non-cross-linked collagen.

New research has shown that the mineral zinc helps minimize the skin eruptions associated with acne. It is theorized that zinc releases vitamin A in the body, which may normalize cells. Another theory is that zinc has anti-inflammatory properties. Both zinc and vitamin C are important in the production of collagen, the main supportive protein of skin, bone and cartilage.

On the other hand, foods containing iodine, such as iodized salt, turkey and broccoli, seem to aggravate acne problems.

Body Brushing for Health and Beauty

As reported above, the skin is an important organ in the elimination process. And, if not cleaned properly, the very

---

Fountain of Youth Secret No. 14

Dry body brushing will cleanse, stimulate, revitalize and beautify the skin surface and underlying tissues.

---

glands that seek to cleanse the body of toxic poisons and metabolic wastes can become clogged and unable to function.

Dry body brushing is an effective way to clean and stimulate the skin and it has a host of benefits. Dry brushing:

1) effectively removes dead layers of skin and impurities.

2) helps open and keep the pores clean.

3) revitalizes and increases the eliminative capacity of the skin.

4) stimulates the hormone- and oil-producing glands.

5) helps rejuvenate the nervous system by stimulating nerve endings.

Both zinc and vitamin C are important in the production of collagen, the main supportive protein of skin, bone and cartilage.

6) contributes to a healthier muscle tone and a
   better distribution of fat deposits.

7) rejuvenates the complexion.

8) improves general health and helps prevent
   premature aging.

Chart 4-1
Dry Body Massage Tools and Techniques

Brush Selection:

Choose a hand-sized brush made of natural fibers. A brush with a handle on it is preferred if the massages will be self-administered. Avoid nylon or other man-made brushes — they can damage the skin.   It may be desirable to pick a less course brush and increase the coarseness as the vitality of the skin improves.

Brushing Instructions:

1. Two times a day, (upon rising and just before bed) brush each part of the body with a vigorous rotary motion until the skin becomes rosy, warm and glowing. Be careful not to brush too hard.

2. Start with soles of feet, work up legs. Then brush hands, arms, back, abdomen, chest, neck and scalp, in that order.

3. Finish with a warm shower or rub body with a course wet towel to remove dead skin particles. Rub a quality moisturizing lotion (one that contains Sodium PCA) all over the skin.

Additional Suggestions:

1. Wash brush once a week with soap and water to remove impurities.

2. Don't share brush with anyone.

3. Don't brush areas of skin that are irritated, damaged or infected.

9) stimulates and increases blood circulation in all under-lying organs and tissues — especially in the small capillaries of the skin.

Chart 4-1 explains the tools and techniques needed for effective dry body massage.

Fountain of Youth Secret No. 15
Sodium PCA is the body's natural moisturizer and is very effective when applied to the skin.

Protecting and Moisturizing the Skin

Maintaining the normal acid mantle of the skin is important for the prevention of dermatitis and other skin conditions and diseases. Most soaps and detergents are alkaline in nature and disrupt the acid mantle. The hair and skin should be cleansed with products that have a pH of six or less. Gloves should be worn when hands might be exposed to household detergents, cleaners, solvents and other caustic chemicals.

Skin cells, as well as the other cells in the body, require large amount of water in order to function properly. In order to help supplement their need for water, skin tissues contain a compound called sodium PCA. Sodium PCA is a sodium salt of 2-pyrrolidone-5-carboxylic acid and is a powerful moisture magnet (a humectant) created by the body.

Skin cells, as well as the other cells in the body, require large amounts of water in order to function properly.

As people age, their bodies produce less and less of this natural moisturizer. Older people have about 50 percent less sodium PCA in their skin than young people, which contributes to skin that feels dry and hard. Topically applied sodium PCA

Chart 4-2
Selecting Skin Care Products

Ingredients to avoid	Reason
Alcohol	Can dry and irritate skin.
Artificial Fragrances	Can produce allergic reactions.
Artificial Colors	Can produce allergic reactions.
Mineral Oil/ Petroleum products	Sits on skin surface and blocks pores.

Animal Proteins
  Collagen
  Elastin
  Placenta
	These substances have extra large molecules which cannot pass through the pores in the skin. They are expensive ingredients which provide no discernable benefit.

Formaldehyde	Used to preserve dead animals, can be harmful to living tissues.

Ingredients to Seek	Reason
Jojoba	Similar to body's own oils — conditions and lubricates skin.
Aloe	Lubricates and moisturizes skin.
Allantoin	Soothing and calming.
Glycerine	Natural humectant/moisturizer.
Panthenol	Aids in cell renewal.
Sodium PCA	Natural humectant/moisturizer.
Tocopherol (Vit. E)	Natural moisturizer, preservative and anti-oxidant.
Retinol (Vit. A)	Natural moisturizer and anti-oxidant.

Natural Plant Oils
  Peanut Oil
  Almond Oil
  Sesame Oil
  Apricot Seed Oil
  Safflower Oil
  Wheat Germ Oil
  Olive Oil
  Avocado Oil
	Rich in biological substances — lock in skin's natural secretions.

(also known as Na-PCA) has been demonstrated to be highly effective as a natural moisturizer.

Animal fats and oils, when applied to the skin, hold in moisture but also clog pores and have been shown to make the skin less supple. Animal proteins like collagen, elastin, and placenta appear in "miracle" creams but are not likely to do much for the skin. The molecules of these protein products are much larger than the pores of the skin and do not penetrate the skin's surface. (See Chart 4-2 for tips on selecting skin care products.)

Footnotes

1. Durk Pearson and Sandy Shaw, *Life Extension* (New York, Warner Books), 1982

Chapter 5

Superfoods and Enzymes

The Power for Life and Living

Enzymes are the powerful building blocks of a healthy life. With them, life can be full of vigor and vitality. Without them, life span is shortened and the body is robbed of precious energy. Superfoods are the substances that contain the highest levels of live enzymes in the plant kingdom.

Nobel Laureate James Sumner of Cornell University defines life as "an orderly functioning of enzymes." Life ends when the worn-out enzyme activity of the body drops to such a low point that it is unable to carry on vital enzyme reactions. The goal is to delay the lessening of enzyme activity. By doing so, years can be added to the life span. What is now called "old age" can actually be transformed into the prime time of life.

The length of life is directly proportional to the enzyme potential in the body. The increased intake of food enzymes increases the enzyme potential of the body and adds to the enzyme reserves. This decreases the rate at which the body must manufacture its own enzymes for metabolic functions, and leaves an abundant supply for disease-fighting and longevity-increasing functions. By eating foods with the enzymes intact, the abnormal and pathological aging processes can be stopped.[1]

Enzymes are the energy-producing building blocks of all life. Life span is directly linked to the enzyme levels in the body.

Why Enzymes Are So Important

Enzymes are essential for maintaining proper functions of the body, digesting food, and aiding in the repair of tissue. Found in all living plants and animals, thousands of known enzymes play a role in virtually all body activities. Life itself could not be sustained without enzymes, despite the presence of sufficient amounts of vitamins, minerals, water and proteins.

Enzymes are needed for beauty, positive attitude, strength, endurance and natural weight normalization. They are also needed to power the immune system and slow down aging.

Enzymes are critical to energy, beauty, positive attitude, physical strength and stamina, decreased need for sleep, and natural weight normalization. They slow down cross-linking, peroxidation, and other aging processes, especially on the cellular and cardiovascular levels. They promote optimum sexuality, and are used by the immune system for targeting and destroying invaders and errant cells. They promote deep cleansing on the cellular level. It's been well said that clean cells are healthy cells.

Characteristics of Enzymes

The body gets enzymes from two sources: from food as well as producing them itself. Enzymes are needed for every bodily function, and it is important that the enzyme production process, which occurs mostly in the liver, not be overloaded. It is equally important that enough enzyme-rich food or supplements be ingested to increase the body's supply.

For example, if the body needs enzymes for digestion of a large meal, other enzymes needed for metabolic function may not be available. The typical low-enzyme diet of the average American uses up a tremendous amount of the body's resources as it struggles to provide the enzymes needed for metabolic activity. Overuse of the body's enzyme production capabilities leaves precious little, if any, enzyme resources left over for disease-fighting and health-maintaining processes.

Enzymes are a miracle in and of themselves. Each one has a specific function that no other enzyme can accomplish. Even the shape of the enzyme molecule is very specialized so that it only reacts with certain other substances.

Enzymes are very susceptible to heat, and even moderate temperatures will destroy them. To get the best enzyme supply from food, it must be eaten raw. Cooked food is depleted of most, if not all, enzymes. It simply does not have the live enzyme activity that our bodies need for proper metabolic and health-giving functions.

Enzymes are destroyed in the range between 118 and 149 degrees fahrenheit. Long heating at 118 degrees, or short heating at 149 degrees, kills enzymes.[2] Water used to cook food typically reaches 180-212 degrees. Therefore most, if not all, the enzymes in these cooked foods are "dead" and of no use to the body. Most normal food processing destroys enzymes and renders them useless. So, if we don't eat raw food, we must take enzyme supplements. To do otherwise is to place a great strain on our bodies.

Bodily production of enzymes also declines as the body ages. This causes an even lower amount of available enzymes. Most foods in the American diet are low in enzymes, and most have enzyme-antagonists in them. It's a vicious cycle. All this further aggravates the situation — enzyme production and bio-availability drops to a low level. The immune and cardiovascular-cardiorespiratory systems are the hardest hit by this low-enzyme condition.

Results of a Low Enzyme Condition

Over 4,000 people in America die every day from heart disease or cancer related deaths. Once enzyme balance is lost, it is very difficult, if not impossible, to gain it back. Enzyme-active foods or supplements help eliminate this dreadful situation, while at the same time greatly improving the quality of life.

Enzymes are the only nutrients that supply the body with energy. Lack of a sufficient supply can impair the functioning of the body, making it susceptible to conditions of ill health such as cancer, obesity, cardiovascular problems, and many other problems.

The majority of supplements available are digestive enzymes, and deal solely with the digestive process. Metabolic enzymes deal with other phases of life processes. All of the

Heat, age, and enzyme-antagonists destroy enzymes and render them useless.

Although the body's need for enzymes remains constant, it produces fewer and fewer enzymes as it grows older.

body's organs, tissues, and cells are run by the metabolic nutrients needed for cells. They are the catalysts for cellular activity.

Coenzyme Q10 is perhaps the single most important enzyme that can be supplemented. Of the metabolic enzymes, superoxide dismutase (SOD) and glutathione peroxidase are two of the most important. SOD and coenzyme Q10 are so important that they are discussed at length in the antioxidant chapter (Chapter Six).

Glutathione peroxidase is also a very important enzyme. Made in the body as well as being ingested from food sources, it is an antioxidant that destroys the free radical electrons. Humans would die without glutathione peroxidase and SOD. Interestingly, each molecule of glutathione peroxidase must contain four atoms of selenium to be effective. Selenium is also discussed in Chapter Six. The relationship between glutathione peroxidase and selenium is but one more indicator of the symbiotic relationship that exists in the body.

It is interesting that enzyme supplementation produced the greatest increase in athletic performance in athletes that were older than 30 years of age. Coincidentally, it is at about this age that the bodily production of enzymes begins to decline. If 30-year old athletes needed and benefited from enzyme supplementation, how much more does the average person need and will benefit from adding live enzyme supplements or superfoods to the daily intake.

Foods to Eat for Enzyme Supplementation

Thus far, more than 3,000 enzymes have been identified. It is possible to get 1,000 of these life-giving, energy-powering enzymes in a single food, as discussed in the superfoods section in this chapter. Low enzyme levels can be improved or eliminated entirely, providing an abundance of power and energy.

Raw foods that contain high amounts of enzymes are avocados, bananas and mangos. Sprouts are the very highest source of enzymes. When buying digestive supplements, look

Impaired enzymatic systems expose the body to cancer, heart and lung problems, and overweight conditions.

for such names as pancreatin, pepsin, and aspergillus. To properly feed and supply the cells, a broad range of nutrients and micro-nutrients is necessary. Single nutrient supplementation may or may not be effective — a full spectrum superfood should be the starting point in the nutritional arsenal against ill health and premature aging.

Superfoods

Superfoods are a special category of enzyme and nutrient-rich foods. They include the wheat and barley grasses (part of the cereal grass family), spirulina, kelp, brown rice, alfalfa, chlorophyll and chlorella. The cereal grasses, rice, and alfalfa

---

Fountain of Youth Secret No. 16
The Diet can be easily supplemented with the important, life-energizing enzymes: Q10 and SOD

---

are land grown, while spirulina, kelp, and chlorella are harvested from the ocean.

Superfoods have been used by humans for thousands of years. They are quite powerful in their nutritional makeup. It is for this reason that they have been cultivated and used by man for centuries. The Egyptians grew wheat grass as one of their staple foods as early as 5000 B.C. Even today, ancestors of those early wheat grass plants still grow along the Nile River.

Yet, with almost 7000 years of growing history behind them, it was only about 50 years ago that biologists made an important discovery. And that discovery is this — when the cereal plant is young, it looks similar in appearance to an ordinary blade of grass. The plant is very leafy, and dark green in color. If left to grow and mature, it will become a stalk of grain and find its way into the food products humans eat. But researchers found that, at this very young age, the plant contains many times the levels of vitamins, minerals, and proteins found in the mature plant. Young wheat grass contains almost 3 times the protein of whole wheat flour, almost 4 times as much fiber, about 7 times as much calcium, 51 times as much vitamin C, 543 times as much chlorophyll, and 23,136 times as much vitamin A. This young plant is a storehouse of enzyme and growth activity.

Cereal Grass Superfoods

Wheat and barley grass, the most common superfood cereal grasses, are a dark leafy green vegetable. A miniscule 5 grams surpasses the nutritional value of spinach in protein, fiber, and iron. Most dietary guidelines suggest five or more servings daily of dark leafy green vegetables. Wheat and barley grass superfoods provide a convenient and tasty way to supplement the diet with much needed nutrients. Wheat and barley grass are general nutrient tonics. They are very

CHART 5-1
Nutrient Comparison (per 100 grams of weight)

Nutrient	Wheat Grass	Whole Wheat Flour
Protein (gm)	32	13
Total dietary fiber (gm)	37	10
Carbohydrates (gm)	37	71
Vitamin A (IU)	23,136	0
Chlorophyll (mg)	543	4
Iron (mg)	34	4
Calcium (mg)	277	41
Vitamin C (mg)	51	0
Folic Acid (mcg)	100	38
Niacin (mg)	6.1	4.3
Riboflavin (mg)	2.03	.12

cleansing and purifying to the body and support an improved sense of well being.

Some superfood formulas give you the coenzyme Q10 equivalent of 130 pounds of raw broccoli daily. And wheat

---

Fountain of Youth Secret No. 17
Superfoods provide dozens of essential proteins, minerals, vitamins, and life-enhancing enzymes

---

grass tablets provide more beta carotene than any other dark green leafy vegetable. Quite simply, it's the best food source for beta carotene known to man.

The soluble minerals and trace elements in superfoods raise the overall energy of the body. They displace toxins and provide valuable nutritional resources. Of the more than 3000 enzymes discovered and identified, it is believed that wheat and barley grass contain up to 1,000 of these life-giving substances. Loaded with thousands of live enzymes, wheat and barley grass superfoods are bustling with growth activity.

One-third of all the known enzymes in the world are in superfoods

Wheat and barley grass are good superfoods to eat. And they are so convenient. Available in both powders and tablets, it is quick, simple and easy to eat complete servings of dark green leafy vegetables throughout the day. Generally, 1 teaspoon of powder or 7 tablets equals 1 serving of vegetables.

Through new manufacturing processes, two companies have developed very good tasting cereal grass-based superfood powders. Mixed with orange juice, they both taste quite good. And since the superfood blend is normally alkaline, it counteracts the acidity in citrus juices. Orange juice tastes much smoother, and grapefruit juice tastes almost as sweet as regular orange juice. The superfood adds a slight mango-like taste for a very satisfying drink.

Barley grass also has the one of the highest natural levels of SOD in the plant kingdom. The Cancer Chemotherapy Center in Tokyo found that one component in green barley juice inhibited the growth of cancer.

Doctors Talk About Superfoods

Dr. Hagiwara of Japan states that, "The leaves of the cereal grasses provide the nearest thing to the perfect food that this planet offers. I have come to believe that the true medicine is young green barley and wheat leaves which are eaten by human beings as staple food... Such grasses as barley, wheat, rye, and rice too are as indispensable as the elements are."[3]

Dr. Ann Wigmore, an early proponent of superfoods, uses a wheatgrass juice with much success. She reports that the

---

CHART 5-2
Beta Carotene Content of Green Foods

Vegetable	Serving Size	IU per Serving	IU per 100 Grams
Dehydrated Cereal Grass	5 Grams (.175 oz.)	1,156	23,136
Carrots (raw)	1/2 cup	6,050	11,000
Kale (raw, finely chopped)	1/2 cup	4,565	8,300
Spinach (raw, finely chopped)	1/2 cup	2,230	7,964
Summer Squash	1/2 cup	410	390
Broccoli (raw, finely chopped)	1/2 cup	680	877
Cabbage (raw, finely chopped)	1/2 cup	60	133

From CEREAL GRASS, WHAT'S IN IT FOR YOU,
Edited by Ronald L. Seibold, M.S.

wheatgrass used in her programs even contains laetrile and abscisic acid, both of which have been believed to have anti-cancer benefits.

Dr. Chiu Nan Lai, University of Texas Health Sciences Center, Houston, Texas, presented information at a meeting of the American Chemical Society which suggested that wheat grass may have cancer preventive properties. Using the standard Ames test, she showed that extracts of wheat grass,

---

CHART 5-3
Typical analysis of 1 serving (7 tablets) of cereal grass

VITAMINS:

Vitamin A	1750 I/U
Vitamin K	280 mcg.
Vitamin C	11 mg.
Vitamin E	1.1 mcg.
Thiamin	10 mcg.
Choline	1 mg.
Riboflavin	71 mcg.
Pyridoxine	45 mcg.
Vitamin B12	1 mcg.
Niacin	263 mcg.
Pantothenic	84 mcg.
Biotin	4 mcg.
Folic Acid	38 mcg.

MINERALS

Calcium	18 mg.
Phosphorus	18 mg.
Potassium	112 mg.
Magnesium	3.6 mg.
Iron	3 mg.
Manganese	35 mg.
Selenium	3.5 mcg.
Sodium	1 mg.
Iodine	7 mcg.
Copper	02 mcg.
Cobalt	1.75 mcg.

PROTEIN	800 mg.
CRUDE FIBER	600 mg.
CALORIES	10
CHLOROPHYLL	19 mg.
CARBOHYDRATES	1.3 gm.

AMINO ACIDS

Lysine	29 mg.
Histidine	16 mg.
Arginine	39 mg.
Aspartic Acid	78 mg.
Threonine	37 mg.
Glutamic Acid	85 mg.
Proline	33 mg.
Glycine	41 mg.
Alanine	48 mg.
Valine	44 mg,
Isoleucine	41 mg.
Leucine	57 mg.
Tyrosine	18 mg.
Phenylalanine	38 mg.
Methionine	15 mg.
Cystine	8 mg.
Tryptophan	4 mg.
Amide	10 mg.
Purines	2 mg.
Serine	85 mg.

From CEREAL GRASS, WHAT'S IN IT FOR YOU,
Edited by Ronald L. Seibold, M.S.

when applied to known carcinogens, decreased their cancer-causing ability by up to 99 percent. [4]

"Foods are the perfect preventive medicine agents. They provide a steady, but low-level amount of non-toxic therapeutic factors over a lifetime . . . varieties of factors that prevent many diseases simultaneously. As a disease preventive, a whole food is often better than individual compounds squeezed out of it . . . a food is a complex bundle of some ten thousand chemicals, breaking it down may simply dissipate its powers." [5]

The U.S Surgeon General has stated, "As the diseases of nutritional deficiency have diminished, they have been replaced by diseases of dietary excess and imbalance — problems that now rank among the leading causes of death in the United States, touch the lives of most Americans, and generate substantial health care costs." [6]

Superfoods and Weight Loss

For many people, an overweight condition is caused by overeating, brought on by the body's attempt to get needed

---

CHART 5-4

One Bottle of a Superfood Formula Provides:

1. High levels of chlorophyll, enzymes, vitamins, and amino acids

2. The same antioxidant activity as 30,800 tablets of S.O.D.

3. As much algal carotene potency factor as 360 natural beta carotene capsules.

4. The Q10 equivalent of 2 tons of raw broccoli.

5. The soluble fiber equivalent of 30 medium apples.

6. A formulated base of kelp and brown rice for maximum nutrient assimilation.

7. Millions of units of antioxidant enzymes, such as cytochrome oxidase, catalases, glutathione peroxidase, methione reductase, and many more.

nutrients. The more food that is eaten without satisfying the body's craving for vitamins, minerals and enzymes, the more hunger signals the body sends. One solution to this never-ending cycle is to provide the body with the needed nutrients. Superfoods have just what the body needs that many Americans are missing in their diets. As superfoods are ingested, the body is satisfied, and hunger cravings subside. Hunger strikes less often, less is eaten, and weight slowly but steadily normalizes. Then, a healthy lifestyle can emerge as more energy becomes available.

Many people report that it has been quite easy for them to lose weight without any dieting simply by providing their body with the superfood nutrients.

CHART 5-5
Cereal Grass Utilization

People with the following conditions have used cereal grasses successfully:

- Acne

- Allergies

- Anemia

- Asthma

- Blood sugar problems

- Constipation — high fiber content

- Diabetes

- Eczema

- Fibromysitis

- Heartburn

- Heart problems

- Low energy levels — some people report having the energy they had as a young person.

- Multiple Sclerosis

- Overweight — great as part of a balanced weight loss program

- Psoriasis

- Weak immune system

Many people report that it has been quite easy for them to lose weight without any dieting simply by providing their body with the superfood nutrients.

More Superfood Benefits

The benefits of an increased fiber diet are now known. Juicing, a current fad, takes a lot of fruit to get juice, and the pulp and fiber is thrown away. It can take up to 50 pounds of

---

CHART 5-6

Some of the Benefits Ascribed to Superfood Supplementation

- Increases ambition

- Increases positiveness

- Increases athletic performance

- Increases energy level and lowers fatigue — some people report having the energy they had as a young person

- Improves complexion

- Normalizes weight

- Helps reduce cholesterol

- Lowers risk for cancer

- Promotes deep cellular nourishment and cleansing

- Builds immune resistance

- Provides resistance to chemical carcinogens

- Provides nutrients essential for normal bone development

- Provides nutrients required for normal function of sight, smell, hearing, taste

- High in B6, B12, vitamin C, iron, calcium, protein

- Provides nutrients required for synthesis of RNA and DNA

- Supports normal fertility in both males and females

- Liquifies solid cholesterol

- Stimulates healing

- Enhances sexual response

- Helps control appetite — Helped one person to "kick" a $150 a month soda pop and ice cream craving

- Promotes weight loss naturally by feeding the body needed nutrients

- Increases circulation

- Enhances oxygenation

- Revitalizes aging cells

- Increases mental efficiency

- Helps to stop free radical cells from damaging the body

- Improves sleep

- Helps relieve allergies

- Lessens allergic reactions

produce per week for a family of four to get one glass of juice a day. Plus, it takes time for juicing and more time for the laborious cleanup.

Superfoods provide all the benefits of juicing with none of the problems and expense.

The antioxidant properties of the superfoods help protect from sidestream cigarette smoke, toxins and free radicals in coffee, and help relieve allergy symptoms, hip pains, sleeplessness, and fibromysitis. Others report increased energy, relief from heartburn, and a more vigorous, youthful appearance. Some users state that their energy level returned to that of their youth. Many adults have reported wonderful benefits from a regular diet of superfoods.

Superfoods revitalize and energize aging cells, stimulate the healing process, increase mental efficiency, and lower the risk of cancer through their carotene components. Some multiple sclerosis patients even report good results from using superfoods.

Alfalfa

Alfalfa, another land-grown superfood, can help pituitary imbalance, detoxify the body, help glands, liver, kidneys, bowels, stomach, and colon. It has been used for whooping cough and to stop colic in babies. Since it assists in the healing of injured mucous membranes, it is said to be helpful in the healing of aneurisms or swelling of arteries.

Alfalfa is very nutritive. It's a great source of vitamins — vitamins A, B2, B6, C, E and K. It is also contains high amounts of minerals — iron, calcium, silicon, magnesium, phosphorus and potassium. Alfalfa may be the most natural aid to calcium assimilation as it contains all the materials needed for calcium utilization by the body. Some report that it has a way of correcting osteoporosis. It also contains protease which helps to digest proteins. Since it alkalizes the body, some people report relief from arthritis.

Superfoods provide all the benefits of juicing with none of the problems and expense.

Spirulina and Chlorella

Spirulina is a sea vegetable with chromium, selenium (antioxidant), fatty acids (GLA and Omega 3), B12, chlorophyll, carotenes, amino acids, antioxidant enzymes, and vitamins and minerals.

Spirulina and chlorella are the water-based superfoods. Spirulina and juice can be sole source nutrition for the body. Some scientists have lived on it for over fifteen years. It's an excellent source of a rare carbohydrate called rhamnose. This carbohydrate is highly favored by athletes for exceptional stamina. Similar types of carbohydrates can be found in chlorella.

Other plant carbohydrates in the superfood family, such as those found in wheat and barley grass, are renowned for the power and stamina that they provide. A spirulina-type food was the major food source for the mighty Aztec civilization centuries ago.

Spirulina contains huge amounts of chlorophyll, good amounts of all the beneficial trace elements, protein, amino acids, vitamins, minerals, essential fats, carbohydrates, carotene, and is a rich source of antioxidant enzymes.

The mighty Aztec civilization lived almost exclusively on a spirulina-type superfood.

CHART 5-7
Studied Uses for Chlorophyll

• High blood pressure	• Radiation
• Obesity	• Wound treatment
• Gastritis	• Body odors
• Ulcers	• Tissue necrosis
• Pancreas and liver problems	• Burns
	• Intestinal disorders
• Cancer	• Colostomy patients

Chlorophyll

Chlorophyll is found in all the green superfoods. It provides the resources needed for the body to build effective red blood cells for strength, energy, and endurance. It's an enzymatic substance found in wheat and barley grass as well as spirulina. It has a molecular structure similar to hemoglobin. One health writer even calls it "liquid oxygenated sunshine."

It is due to this similarity that chlorophyll, over the years, has attained a reputation as a "blood builder." Components of chlorophyll found in foods help to stimulate the synthesis of red blood cells in the bone marrow. It provides the resources that are essential for building healthy red blood cells for strength, energy, and endurance.

It is high in the antioxidant enzymes such as superoxide dismutase (SOD), glutathione peroxidase, methione reductase, catalases and cytochrome oxidase. All these enzymes neutralize toxic compounds in the body before they can inflict serious damage. And as we've already discussed, longevity and increased life span is relative to the amount of elimination of free radical electrons from the body.

Kelp, enzymes, garlic, and protein amino acids have been used for years to help withstand the common cold virus.

These same nutrients also help to elevate the body's immune system by supplying needed enzymes and trace elements.

Footnotes

1. Dr. Edward Howell, *Enzyme Nutrition* (New Jersey, Avery Publishing), 1985

2. Howell, *Enzyme Nutrition*

3. Dr. Yoshihide Hagiwara, *Green Barley Essence* (Connecticut, Keats Publishing), 1985

4. C. Lai, B. Dabney, and C. Shaw, "Inhibition of in vitro metabolic activation of carcinogens of wheat sprout extracts" *Nutrition and Cancer*, 1978,

5. John Naisbitt, "The Healing Power of Food", *New Age*, 1985

6. "Surgeon General's Report on Nutrition and Health, July 27, 1988, Summary and Recommendation", *Nutrition Today*, Sept. 1988

Chapter 6

Antioxidants and Anti-Aging

Antioxidants are those nutrients that seek out and rid the body of free radical electrons. As discussed in Chapter One, free radicals can be created by the natural processes of the body, as well as by foreign matter, chemicals, and inhaled gases. Even the process of breathing causes trillions of free radical electrons to be released every minute. As oxygen is inhaled, it robs other molecules of an electron. The resulting free-floating electron is the dangerous free radical.

Normally, the body can produce enough antioxidants to combat these particles. The problems start when free radical electrons outnumber the body's antioxidants. This happens normally as a result of aging, and can be aggravated by pollution, smoking, or other toxins. If left to themselves, free radicals roam the body seeking to merge with another electron. In so doing, they create more and more free radicals. Healthy cells are damaged when these free radicals steal electrons from them. Thus, free radicals have been linked to many diseases, among them cancer, osteoarthritis, atherosclerosis, high blood pressure, Alzheimer's disease, and immune deficiency.

Antioxidants are critical, then, to normal body function. They eliminate free radicals created during the course of normal cellular activity.

Gladys Block, School of Public Health, University of California, Berkeley, examined a large number of studies looking at the relationship between fruit and vegetable intake

Antioxidants neutralize free radicals, which have been linked to many diseases such as cancer, arthritis, high blood pressure, & atherosclerosis

Longevity depends on the amount of antioxidant reserves left over after normal cell function has taken place.

and cancer. She found that eating more fruits and vegetables could cut the risk of getting certain kinds of cancers in half. Her review, published in the Journal of Nutrition and Cancer, overwhelmingly shows that high fruit and vegetable consumption has a protective effect against many kinds of cancer. "For practically every cancer, there's impressive evidence that the nutrients in fruits and vegetables work to help lower a person's risk of getting the disease."

Fruits in particular were significantly protective in cancers of the esophagus, oral cavity, and larynx. Fruits and vegetables had a protective effect in cancers of the pancreas, stomach, colorectal, and bladder tissues. Americans have grown up knowing that they should take more vitamin C or eat oranges if they have a cold, and that they should eat more vegetables. Fruits and vegetables are the main source of nutrients that are classified as antioxidants. (Green superfoods are considered to be vegetables.)

Longevity and healing energy is dependent on the reserves of antioxidant resources left over after all the vital cell functions in the body have been accomplished. If the bodily supply of antioxidants are utilized to maintain the body's functions on a cellular level, there will be little or nothing left to maintain, build, and improve energy levels and cellular free radical protection. That may mean an artificially shortened life span, and decreased life enjoyment due to lowered energy levels. With all the impressive benefits of the antioxidant supplements, this chapter will discuss each one.

Beta Carotene and Vitamin A

The body's own systems defend it from cancer cells thousands of times each day. It performs this task by recombining certain food resources into a substance scientists call "tumor necrosis factor-alpha." It uses this alpha factor to specifically target and dissolve cancer cells without killing normal cells or producing side-effects. Many believe that the scientific data indicates that beta carotene and vitamin A may well be the most important substance for this process.

Dr. Sheldon Hendler says, "There are literally hundreds of papers demonstrating that vitamin A can suppress the malignancy of cultured cells transformed by radiation, chemicals, or viruses, delay the development of transplanted

---

Fountain of Youth Secret No. 17
Natural beta carotene supplementation is an important nutritional weapon in the anti-aging arsenal

---

tumors, and completely prevent malignancy in animals exposed to various potent carcinogens." [1]

The American Cancer Society says that "Foods rich in beta carotene may lower your risk of cancer." [2]

The scientific evidence is mounting that beta carotene can reduce occurrence of a number of forms of cancer. The National Academy of Sciences states "The epidemiological evidence is sufficient to suggest that foods rich in carotene or vitamin A are associated with a reduced risk of cancer." [3]

There are two types of vitamin A — preformed or active, (usually called retinol or vitamin A), and the provitamin carotenoids (beta carotene). Preformed A is found in animal sources like liver, fish, and eggs. It is an oil-soluble compound, and as such, can build up in the body to undesirable levels.

The carotenoid form is found in plants like yellow fruits, yellow vegetables, and dark green leafy vegetables. The body takes preformed beta carotene and converts only as much as it needs to vitamin A. Therefore, it cannot build up to such high undesirable levels like the oil-soluble vitamin A can. Beta carotene is a safe source of high amounts of provitamin A. As beta carotene intake increases, the body converts only what it

Vitamin A and beta carotene are proven cancer fighters, but beta carotene is water-soluble, and can be taken in higher amounts than vitamin A for maximum antioxidant effect.

needs, and the conversion extent to vitamin A decreases. Beta carotene can be taken without undue concern for toxicity.

Vitamin A increases longevity in people — beta carotene is the best source of provitamin A.

Both forms of vitamin A are effective in maintaining healthy eyes and skin. And it is required for the maintenance and growth of teeth, nails, hair, bones, and glands. But the most important benefit is its antioxidant effect. Only the carotenoid beta carotene form serves as an antioxidant in the body. And since beta carotene does not build up in the body, it can be taken in higher amounts to get the most antioxidant effect. The most potent antioxidants are those naturally occurring in beta carotene, vitamins C and E, and the trace mineral selenium.

Vitamin A levels have been demonstrated to be proportional to longevity in mammals. It cleans the cells, and clean cells are high energy cells. It is critical to normal body function. Beta carotene/vitamin A helps eliminate free radicals created during the course of normal cellular activity.

Since the release of the research data showing the efficacy of beta carotene as a cancer fighter, many Americans have sought to add it to their diet, naturally or through supplementation. It can be found in convenience stores, department stores, drug stores, and vitamin centers all over the country. For the most part however, what is being purchased is a synthetic. The question is, "Does synthetic or algal carotene best trigger the body's natural defense mechanisms?"

Synthetic antioxidant beta carotene is obtained from petroleum derivatives, and contains sugar, gelatin, food starch, coconut oil, methylparaben, propylparaben, ascorbyl palmitate, sodium bisulfite, sodium benzoate, butylated hydroxyanisole, residues from chemical intermediates, and hexane solvent residue. The average storage time from finished product to consumer is eighteen months. In spite of all the above chemicals, these types of products are many times labeled as "natural" or "beta carotene."

Synthetic beta carotene does not provide the alpha factor that natural beta carotene does. Harvard University professors Dr. Schwartz and Dr. Shklar studied synthetic versus natural beta carotene. Natural beta carotene was found to be almost eight times more potent than synthetic beta carotene.

Chart 6-1 clearly shows that natural beta carotene is more powerful than synthetic beta carotene. Beta carotene supplementation, or eating foods high in beta carotene, is an important part of an anti-aging plan.

Foods rich in beta carotene are carrots, asparagus, broccoli, brussel sprouts, cabbage, cantaloupe, cauliflower, spinach, sweet potatoes, and turnips. The most potent source of natural beta carotene is an ocean-grown superfood called dunaliella salina.

Both government and consumer surveys have shown that many Americans are not receiving sufficient amounts of vitamin A and other essential nutrients, even though they may appear to have an adequate diet. Cruciferous vegetables, such as broccoli and cauliflower, are good sources of beta carotene. Unfortunately, these are the vegetables that are eaten least. It is now possible to get the beta carotene equivalent of over 1 ton of broccoli in easy-to-take supplements. Beta carotene, coupled

Harvard University found that natural beta carotene is almost 8 times more effective than synthetic beta carotene.

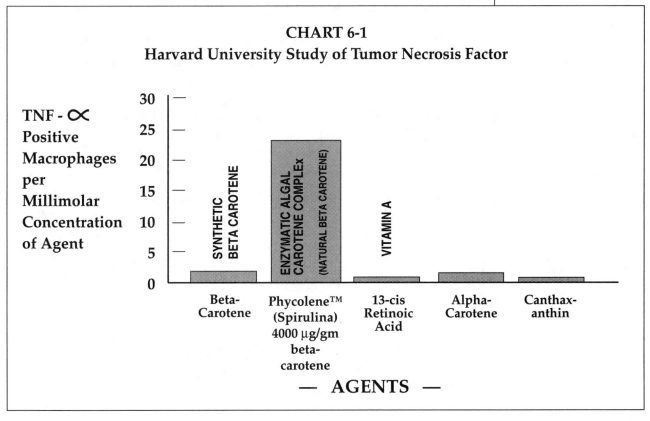

CHART 6-1
Harvard University Study of Tumor Necrosis Factor

6-5

with superfoods and Q10 supplementation, provides an incredible defense against premature aging and the diseases that accompany it.

There is always a substantial amount of oxidation underway in the lungs. Beta carotene protects both the mucous lining and the red blood cells that pass through the lungs and pick up their loads of oxygen for delivery to the cells.

Beta carotene protects the lungs, red blood cells, and may be an Alzheimer's Disease preventative.

Recent studies have linked low blood level of vitamin A and beta carotene to Alzheimer's. Since beta carotene supplementation raises the blood levels of vitamin A, this supplement may also be an Alzheimer's disease preventative. Both vitamin A and beta carotene are antioxidants that help thwart the effects of aging. Note that nutrients from capsules

---

CHART 6-2
Benefits of Maintaining High Levels of
Beta Carotene in the Body

- Better health from resistance to disease.

- Essential for good skin and vision.

- Acts as a powerful antioxidant — helps eliminate free radicals caused by smoking and eating dark roasted foods (coffee) and from radiation therapy.

- Keeps skin, eyes, and the inner linings of the body healthy and resistant to infection.

- May help control/defeat Alzheimer's disease.

- Helps prevent cancer.

- Boosts immune system

- Essential in the maintenance and growth of teeth, nails, hair, bones, and glands.

- Protects against photosensitivity by sunlight.

- It's a non-toxic form of provitamin A, so there's little concern about over-supplementation.

---

are more fully utilized by the bodies of older people than nutrients from natural sources. [4]

The need for many vitamins may increase during periods of stress or illness. And finicky eaters and children may miss out on some of the vitamin content from foods that they don't like to eat. It would be wise to consider additional beta carotene supplementation for any of these situations.

Lung and throat cancer from smoking have been linked to a lack of beta carotene and vitamin B-complex. Drinking fresh carrot juice daily is a good preventative against lung cancer. But a good natural beta carotene supplement will provide the same protection at a much lower cost.

Lung and throat cancer has been linked to a lack of beta carotene and B-complex vitamins.

Fountain of Youth Secret No. 18
Selenium is a proven cancer fighter, increases antibodies and may protect from cardiovascular disease

---

Selenium

"There is no dispute over selenium's cancer-fighting antioxidant effects" states Dr. Sheldon Hendler. "Population studies show that where this mineral intake is lowest, cancer rates are the highest." [5]

And selenium also appears to be a powerful immune system stimulator. Up to thirty-fold increases in antibody production have been found in animals given both selenium and vitamin E. Cardiovascular disease increases as selenium intake decreases.

Dr. Hendler also points out, "The current Recommended Dietary Allowances simply do not deal with the maximization of life span. In no way are they concerned with the anti-aging or antioxidant properties of nutrients... Within the next twenty years, authorities will recommend increased antioxidant supplementation."[6]

Selenium is a necessary component of the glutathione peroxidase enzyme system that destroys free radical molecules. As was discussed in the enzyme section of Chapter Five, glutathione peroxidase needs four atoms of selenium to be effective. The body's production of this important enzyme depends on selenium. And yet, soil stores of this mineral have been all but depleted. Since Selenium acts as a powerful antioxidant, many antioxidant formulas blend it with other antioxidants, such as vitamin C, beta carotene, and vitamin E into a potent free radical eliminator formula.

There is very little selenium left in our soil. Supplementation is recommended for maximum antioxidant benefits.

Selenium has been demonstrated to be proportional to longevity in mammals. It cleans the cells, and clean cells are high energy cells.

Selenium enhances immunity and inhibits cancer, especially of the digestive tract. It also helps prevent free radical damage from radiation therapy, and helps eliminate the free radicals caused by smoking and eating dark roasted foods (such as coffee).

Vitamin C and Bioflavonoids

Vitamin C is a virtual storehouse of dietary benefits. It acts as an antioxidant, as well as being considered the cornerstone of the vitamin world. Many people only equate vitamin C with being useful for colds and viruses. It has uses far beyond that of only a single-use cold symptom reliever. Vitamin C and the accompanying bioflavonoids have earned their well-deserved reputation as a nutritional cornerstone.

BIOFLAVONOIDS

The bioflavonoids, sometimes called C-complex, were originally called vitamin P by Nobel Laureate discoverer Albert Gyorgyi in 1936. In 1950, biochemist B.L. Oser renamed vitamin P as bioflavonoids.

Bioflavonoids are naturally occurring compounds found primarily in citrus products, but also occurring throughout nature in the plant kingdom. There are three main types: flavones, flavonols, and flavonones.

Fountain of Youth Secret No. 18
Bioflavonoids work with vitamin C to stabilize biological functions

---

Rutin, citrin, and hesperidin are three flavonoids best known for their synergistic effect with vitamin C. Rutin especially is generally accepted as a remedy, in combination with vitamin C, for persistent bleeding, to care for hemorrhoids, and to delay the onset of capillary fragility that usually comes with aging.

Most of the general information that applies to vitamin C also applies to the bioflavonoids. They are non-toxic, readily absorbed into the bloodstream from the intestinal tract, and any excess is eliminated through perspiration or urination. Bioflavonoid deficiencies are much the same as vitamin C deficiencies. An absence of either C or bioflavonoids produces the equivalent result — bleeding and bruising are among the most common symptoms. It is a little known fact that there is a C-complex group which includes bioflavonoids. These two factors, vitamin C and bioflavonoids, work together in stabilizing various biological functions.

Dr. Gyorgyi saw that the lack of bioflavonoids caused cerebral edema and bleeding in Hungary after World War II. Both of these are signs of capillary fragility. Dr. Gyorgyi extracted two different bioflavonoids which appeared to be effective in reducing capillary permeability and lowering resistance to hemorrhaging of the tiny blood vessels.

Bioflavonoid deficiencies are much the same as vitamin C deficiencies — bleeding and bruising are among the most common symptoms.

Capillary resiliency is what permits the delicate function of the inner ear, and is thereby related to hearing and balance. Research in this area has demonstrated that C-complex is a treatment for inner ear malfunctions that occur from weak capillaries.

Other problems linked to vitamin C-bioflavonoid deficiency are habitual miscarriages, hemorrhages, bleeding gums, eczema, and rheumatism. Certain specific problems such as blood vessel disorders, especially of the eyes (common among diabetics), and lowering of blood pressure among muscular dystrophy sufferers have been treated with C and bioflavonoids. C-complex is being tested for the treatment of arteriosclerosis, high cholesterol, hemophilia, leukemia, stroke, arthritis, and ulcers.

The lemon has the highest quantity of bioflavonoids. Fifteen to twenty different ones are found in this fruit. Limes, tangerines, grapefruits, and oranges also have high amounts but not in as wide a spectrum as lemons. All the different types of bioflavonoids have not yet been catalogued, and some have probably not even been discovered. Bioflavonoids remain an important part of the anti-aging arsenal.

VITAMIN C

When vitamin C is processed into a single substance supplement, it loses the bioflavonoids that naturally exist in the source. It is a common practice for the manufacturer to return some of the bioflavonoids to the final vitamin C product, but how much and of what type is up to them. Look for a high quality vitamin C with as many bioflavonoids as possible. Look for bioflavonoid names such as hesperidin, rutin, citrin, naringen, naringenin, eriocitrin, and bilberry.

Studies show that blood levels of vitamin C in smokers are as much as 30 percent lower than in non-smokers. Antioxidants and other nutrients for smokers would consist of an antioxidant blend, B-complex supplementation, vitamin C, beta carotene, zinc, coenzyme Q10, vitamin E, raw thymus, and germanium.

Vitamin A, beta carotene, and vitamin C are helpful to withstand the common cold virus. Zinc and the herb goldenseal have also been effective. Even dieting may reduce levels of vitamin C due to skipping or eliminating the vitamin C rich foods. Vitamin C supplementation is a dietary requirement in today's world.

Linus Pauling recommends large doses. He found that large doses of vitamin C have no harmful side effects. Dr. Hoffer has used daily doses as high as 30,000 mgs. in more than 1,000 patients since 1953 without one case of kidney stone formation, excessive hydration, or any other serious toxicity. [7]

Dr. Klenner has given patients 10,000 mgs. daily for over thirty years without any serious toxic effects. [8]

Vitamin C has been demonstrated to be proportional to longevity in mammals. It cleans the cells, and clean cells are high energy cells.

Smokers need additional vitamin C — smoking depletes up to 30% of the blood level of vitamin C.

Fountain of Youth Secret No. 19
Research shows that the daily addition of 900 mgs. of vitamin C to the diet can add 10 years to human life span.

Vitamin C and Life Extension

The University of California at Los Angeles (UCLA) recently completed a 21 year-long study of the effects of vitamin C supplementation on human longevity. This study was begun in 1971, and analyzed 11,348 adults for their vitamin C intake and general health. The findings of this significant study are absolutely astounding.

First, they proved that men can expect a life-expectancy increase of six years by taking only 500 mgs. of vitamin C daily. Women can expect a one year life span extension using that same dose. And a 900 mg. daily dose of vitamin C results in a

CHART 6-3

UCLA Study of Effects of Vitamin C on Longevity

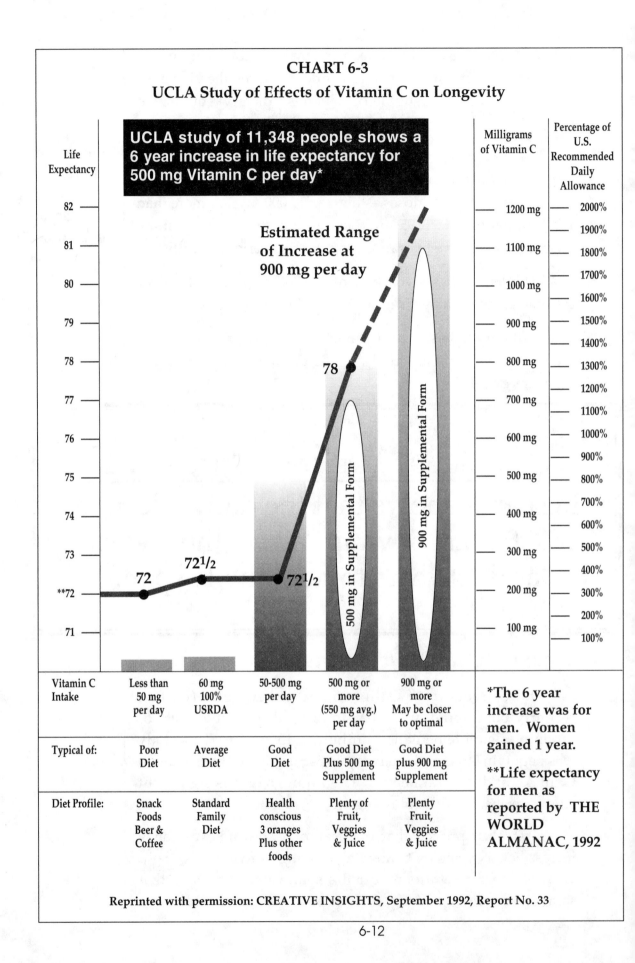

UCLA study of 11,348 people shows a 6 year increase in life expectancy for 500 mg Vitamin C per day*

Estimated Range of Increase at 900 mg per day

Life Expectancy

82
81
80
79
78
77
76
75
74
73
**72
71

72
72 1/2
72 1/2
78

500 mg in Supplemental Form

900 mg in Supplemental Form

Milligrams of Vitamin C

1200 mg
1100 mg
1000 mg
900 mg
800 mg
700 mg
600 mg
500 mg
400 mg
300 mg
200 mg
100 mg

Percentage of U.S. Recommended Daily Allowance

2000%
1900%
1800%
1700%
1600%
1500%
1400%
1300%
1200%
1100%
1000%
900%
800%
700%
600%
500%
400%
300%
200%
100%

Vitamin C Intake	Less than 50 mg per day	60 mg 100% USRDA	50-500 mg per day	500 mg or more (550 mg avg.) per day	900 mg or more May be closer to optimal
Typical of:	Poor Diet	Average Diet	Good Diet	Good Diet Plus 500 mg Supplement	Good Diet plus 900 mg Supplement
Diet Profile:	Snack Foods Beer & Coffee	Standard Family Diet	Health conscious 3 oranges Plus other foods	Plenty of Fruit, Veggies & Juice	Plenty Fruit, Veggies & Juice

*The 6 year increase was for men. Women gained 1 year.

**Life expectancy for men as reported by THE WORLD ALMANAC, 1992

Reprinted with permission: CREATIVE INSIGHTS, September 1992, Report No. 33

life extension of ten years! And they found that men, especially, benefit from vitamin C's preventative influence on heart disease and stress-related disorders. Clearly, vitamin C is more important than most doctors and medical experts realize. And it takes doses far in excess of 60 mgs. per day to get the desired life-extending benefits.

Oranges are the food most quickly associated with vitamin C. They are inexpensive, readily available, and delicious. Other foods rich in vitamin C are citrus fruits, papayas, currants, strawberries, brussel sprouts, green peppers, and cantaloupe or honeydew melons.

Vitamin C and Conditions of Ill Health

It has been demonstrated that vitamin C adds years to human life. It's an antioxidant that slows down the cell damage process from toxins, thereby increasing our life-span. Now it appears that aging has as much to do with the amount of antioxidants in the system as it does with the physical process of time. Vitamin C and other antioxidants will keep people feeling and looking younger than their actual age. And aging exposes the body to the three greatest threats to health — cancer, heart disease, and infections.

The Linus Pauling Institute found in one study that the risk from cancer can be reduced by 80% with adequate intake of vitamin C. Thirty three other studies have found that vitamin C prevents numerous types of cancer. Dr. Eymard Poydock of Mercyhurst College, Erie, Pennsylvania, noted that vitamins C and B12 work together to prevent division of tumor cells without damaging normal cells.

Dr. Melvyn Werbach, M.D., in his book Nutritional Influences on Illness, reported that cholesterol levels dropped 41 points in only 6 weeks after beginning daily doses of 1000 mgs. of vitamin C. This one health tip alone could save the lives of hundreds of thousands of Americans every year.

Dr. Abram Hoffer M.D., in his book Orthomolecular Medicine for Physicians, states that Vitamin C is also effective against infections. It detoxifies bacterial toxins and helps to destroy invading substances.

Thirty three different studies prove that Vitamin C prevents cancer. It is also effective for reducing cholesterol levels, fighting infections and eliminating toxins.

CHART 6-4
Benefits of Maintaining High Levels of Vitamin C in the Body

- Vitamin C increases both the number and quality of white blood cells.

- Blocks the cancer-promoting effects of nitrosamines.

- Some evidence shows that it can suppress the growth of human leukemia cells in culture.

- High doses boost the body's production of interferon, a virus-fighting substance.

- Antioxidant properties.

- Retards aging process.

- Better health from resistance to disease.

- It's water soluble and helps guard the body against harmful reactions within the cell.

- Makes capillaries stronger.

- Delays capillary fragility of the aging process.

- Helps control bleeding and bruising.

- Helps stabilize the inner ear functions.

- Helps restore equilibrium and balance.

- Helps habitual miscarriages, hemorrhages, bleeding gums, eczema and rheumatism.

- Combats effects of low vitamin C in smokers.

- Helps eliminate free radicals caused by smoking and eating dark roasted foods (coffee) and damage from radiation therapy.

- Helps fight cancer

- May have mild anti-viral effects.

- May help arteriosclerosis, high cholesterol, hemophilia, leukemia, stroke, arthritis, and ulcers.

Some people believe that, in general, nutrients are absorbed into the body faster if exposed in a powder or effervescent form to the neural and sublingual receptors under the tongue. Otherwise, a pill must be broken down in the stomach before it can be utilized by the body. This process takes from about 17 minutes to as long as 1-1/2 hours, depending on the condition of the digestive system and food content in the stomach.

An almost immediate utilization is accomplished when vitamins are absorbed in the mouth. Only three companies worldwide have developed effervescent vitamins that are dissolved in water. The tablet or powder is dissolved in a glass of water, and drunk. This is an easy and delicious way to take vitamins.

There is a new antioxidant that is even more powerful than vitamin C called pycnogenol. Fifty mgs. of vitamin. C provide about 50 units of antioxidant potential, whereas 50 mgs. of pycnogenol provides 1000 units of antioxidant potential — 20 times the antioxidant potential. A natural substance from pine trees, pycnogenol is among the most powerful antioxidants known to man.

Bilberry is also an important antioxidant as it is a holder/carrier of vitamin C. Any of these three substances, vitamin C, pycnogenol, or bilberry, make for a powerful antioxidant. And a blend of all three would deliver a staggering knockout punch to free radical invaders. And one biochemist believes that adding bilberry and pycnogenol to vitamin C boosts the antioxidant properties by as much as 3000%.

Vitamin E and Lecithin

An essential nutrient, an adequate vitamin E intake results in a feeling of accomplishment and well-being. Nutritional needs for vitamin E are quite low — about 20 IU daily. Some vitamin E enthusiasts, however, safely take up to 1000 IU daily to get its powerful antioxidant benefits.

The primary function of vitamin E is to maintain the stability of cell membranes and protect them from free radicals

50 mg. of pycnogenol provides 1000 units of antioxidant potential — 20 times the antioxidant potential of Vitamin C.

and peroxidation (oxygen containing compounds). Vitamin E protects fat-containing membranes such as those found in the nerves, muscles, and cardiovascular system. It helps prolong the life of red blood cells, and it also helps the body utilize vitamin A to its fullest. Once more, we see the wonderful synergy of nutrition and the human body.

Vitamin E is an entire family of molecules known as tocopherols. They are broadly classified as either synthetic or natural. While some people maintain that there is no difference between natural and synthetic vitamins, this is not the case with vitamin E. Synthetic vitamin E is very different from natural vitamin E.

D-tocopherols are the natural form, and are "right-handed" in construction. This is how vitamin E exists in nature. The Dl-tocopherols are a mixture of natural and synthetic forms (the "l" indicates synthetic "left-handed" vitamin E). D-tocopherols are more bio-active than the Dl-tocopherols.

The second part of the name for vitamin E can be one of four terms: alpha, beta, gamma, or delta. These are the names for the primary vitamin E forms found in nature. All four forms together most closely resemble the vitamin E found in food sources. The alpha form is the most biologically nutrient active, and the potency of vitamin E is measured in terms of the D-alpha content.

If you see a "-yl" ending to the word, e.g. tocopheryl, it means that the alpha compound has been separated from the other forms by a special process. The "-ol" ending, e.g. tocopherol, is used to indicate that all four vitamin E forms are present, and no isolation has taken place.

The primary food source is seed oils and margarines, and shortenings made from these oils. Nuts, seeds, whole grains (the germ), dark leafy green vegetables, eggs and milk are also good sources.

Wheat germ oil contains much more vitamin E than any other oil — 10 IU in a teaspoon. Highly unsaturated, (about 75%), linoleic acid, the most essential saturated fatty acid is found in wheat germ oil. Because of all these properties, wheat germ oil has been shown to strengthen the heart action, improve efficiency of all muscles, fortify the glands, prevent menopausal symptoms, and enhance fertility and virility.

Fountain of Youth Secret No. 20
Vitamin E feeds the heart, brain & glands with antioxidants and has been used to treat menopausal symptoms.

Some people believe that wheat germ oil possesses a mysterious fat-like substance that all the body's cells use to create prostaglandins, hormones that regulate all the metabolic activities of the body, making certain that the brain, nerves, muscles, glands, organs, and connective tissues work together consistently.

Wheat germ oil is also one of the few oils available that is crude, raw, and unrefined. Most clear golden-looking salad or cooking oils, unless specifically stated otherwise, are refined, bleached, deflavored, and deodorized. Some companies use industrial-type solvents in the refining process for their food oils. Cold-pressed or expeller-pressed oils — a natural process that doesn't use solvents — are much superior. This type of oil is reasonably priced and can now be found in almost all supermarkets and grocery stores.

Wheat germ oil with naturally existing vitamin E is better than vegetable oil with added vitamin E.

In 1972, Dr. Cureton published "The Physiological Effects of Wheat Germ Oil on Humans in Exercise." Controlled experiments show conclusively that vegetable oils with the same added natural vitamin E amount did *not* produce the same results in exercise tolerance as did wheat germ oil. His study of 894 humans showed that octacosanol and other elements in wheat germ oil produced statistically significant improved effects on athletic performance compared to average vegetable oils with added vitamin E.

Dietary deficiency of vitamin E is rare, however vitamin E is an important antioxidant, and most people need additional antioxidant supplementation. Laboratory studies reveal that a lack of vitamin E is associated with shortened red blood cell survival time, muscle loss, increased production of ceroid aging pigment in certain tissues, some genetic blood diseases such as sickle cell anemia and thalassemia. Recent investigations have shown that vitamin E deficiency caused by the liver disorder biliary atresia resulted in a rare type of progressive neuro-muscular disease in children. Symptoms include a loss of coordination and balance, and loss of ability to walk in severe cases.

As an antioxidant, vitamin E intake has been demonstrated to be proportional to longevity in mammals. Antioxidants clean the cells, and clean cells are high energy cells. The most potent antioxidants are naturally occurring beta carotene, vitamins C and E, and the trace mineral selenium.

Researchers at the Mayo Clinic in Minnesota found that vitamin E drastically lowered the number of free radicals in the blood. The recommendation from Dr. Nicholas Cavarocchi was that patients receive a dose of vitamin E, up to 2000 IU, twelve hours before heart surgery. It is known that surgery, especially heart bypass surgery, causes an excess of free radical electrons in the body. Dr. Cavarocchi says that vitamin E could make heart surgery a safer procedure. [9]

Vitamin E is rich in sterols, potent hormones in the body. This is why it's reputed to be very invigorating for the procreative and reproductive organs. In fact, vitamin E is so very important for sexual well-being that it has been called the sex vitamin. It also reinforces the adrenal glands, bringing increased stamina and athletic endurance.

A recent survey at the University of Western Ontario suggested that vitamin E may help prevent cataracts. The researchers found that people who did not have cataracts took significantly higher doses of vitamin E and C than those people with cataracts. Those people who took vitamin E alone had

Recent investigations have shown that vitamin E deficiency caused by a liver disorder resulted in a rare type of progressive neuro-muscular disease in children.

about 1/2 the risk of developing cataracts as those who took no vitamin E. Those who took vitamin E and C had 2/3 fewer cataracts than those people who took neither vitamin. [10]

Studies have also shown promising results among Parkinson's patients who took vitamins E and C. Dr. Stanley Fahn's patients have been able to go for 2-1/2 years longer than other patients before having to resort to potent medicine treatments of levodopa.

In animal testing, vitamin E helps prevent artery clogging from plaque buildup. Without vitamin E, an LDL particle contains only eight to ten antioxidant molecules. These few molecules can only do so much. A higher blood level of vitamin E means fewer free radicals.

In human research at Tufts University, the blood samples of vitamin E-supplemented patients showed a higher level of biochemical immune function. Immune T-cells were healthier and more productive. These immune cells were able to "communicate" better among themselves, which means that they can battle invaders more readily. It is possible that additional research will prove that vitamin E will boost the body's immune system.

A study from Scotland offers preliminary evidence that vitamin E shields lung cells and red blood cells from oxidative damage due to smoking. (The animal study has already shown that it lessens smoke-induced cell damage.) The study included forty people, smokers and non-smokers, who took 1000 IU of vitamin E daily. After only two weeks, the blood cells of smokers were less likely to be damaged by smoking.

Some studies have suggested that vitamin E plays a role in the cellular generation of energy.

A study of 21,172 men in Finland found that those who had high blood levels of vitamin E were less likely to develop cancer than were those with low levels of vitamin E. A similar study with 15,093 women had the same result — vitamin E protects against cancer.

Vitamin E has been shown in animal studies to help protect against damage from environmental pollutants. New evidence

Studies have shown that Vitamin E may prevent cataracts, arterial plaque buildup associated with heart disease, and help Parkinson's Disease patients.

New evidence indicates that vitamin E may have a therapeutic role in fibrocystic breast disease, heart murmurs, premenstrual syndrome (PMS), and progressive neuromuscular disease in children.

indicates that vitamin E may have a therapeutic role in fibrocystic disease of the breast (a possible precursor to breast cancer), intermittent claudication, premenstrual syndrome (PMS), and progressive neuromuscular disease in children.

Lecithin

Lecithin is being widely recommended by some of the world's top medical researchers for a variety of conditions of ill health. Even the medical establishment is baffled as its own members prove that this natural substance can help more and

---

CHART 6-5

Benefits of Maintaining High Levels of
Vitamin E and Lecithin in the Body

- Better health from resistance to disease.

- Vitamin E appears to have anti-blood-clotting effects.

- Adds to selenium's cancer-fighting antioxidant effects..

- Slows down the aging process.

- May improve circulation.

- Relieves leg pain when walking.

- Vitamin E protects the good fatty acids from free radical attack.

- Improves the efficiency of the heart.

- Studies have shown that vitamin E protects against damage from environmental pollutants and cigarette smoke.

- Antioxidant properties help eliminate free radicals caused by smoking and eating dark roasted foods (coffee) and free radical damage from radiation therapy.

---

more brain disorders, as well as heart, liver, and psychiatric disorders.

Dr. Richard Wurtman, M.D., of the Massachusetts Institute of Technology, was among the first researchers who started this new flurry of activity to test lecithin on neurological disorders. His findings proved that the amount of lecithin eaten directly affects the chemical activity of the brain.

According to the medical community, only one of the phosphatides naturally present in lecithin really works for these disorders — phosphatidyl choline. Some lecithins only have about 25% of this component. It is very important to get lecithin with a high value of phosphatidyl choline in it.

West German researchers have found that phosphatidyl choline helps patients with alcoholic, fatty livers. [11]

At the same time, scientists in Prague use phosphatidyl choline on what is medically called "non-biliary, non-alcoholic, micronodular cirrhosis of the liver." This appears to suggest that one can develop cirrhosis even if one doesn't drink alcoholic beverages. Scientists chose subjects who had not responded to treatment for over six months. After six months' treatment with phosphatidyl choline, 26 of the 32 "incurable" patients showed marked improvement, including weight gain,

25% of Alzheimer's patients treated with lecithin showed great improvement

91 patients with high cholesterol counts were fed a high-fat diet with a teaspoon of lecithin at each meal — 79% ended up with lower cholesterol.

CHART 6-6
Food High in Vitamin E and Lecithin

- Sunflower seeds or oil
- Sesame seeds or oil
- Almonds or oil
- Canola, soy, or corn oils
- Wheat germ
- Whole grain products
- Liver
- Dried beans
- Dark green leafy vegetables

---

disappearance of digestive problems, better sleep patterns, loss of fatigue, and decreased psychological problems. A battery of tests established that phosphatidyl choline "improved the structure and metabolism of the damaged liver cells." [12]

Fountain of Youth Secret No. 21

Lecithin dissolves cholesterol, fuels creativity, supports healthy skin and feeds the muscles and brain.

One of the most important neurological disorders on which scientists have been testing phosphatidyl choline is Alzheimer's disease. A study offers very hopeful beginnings to this research. After only eight weeks of treatment with phosphatidyl choline, 25% of the subject patients reported astounding results. One patient, who was so deteriorated that she could not be left home alone safely, was able to "go on errands." One other patient who had suffered great slowing of thought, speech, and movement "has shown a great increase in fluency so that she is more alert and effective in social interaction." [13]

Lecithin also helps prevent heart disease and is used to treat already existing arteriosclerosis. Dr. Francis Pottenger, M.D., took 91 patients who already had high cholesterol counts, fed them a high-fat diet with a teaspoon of lecithin at each meal. 79% ended up with lower cholesterol. [14]

Lecithin is the finest practical source of essential fatty acids available. After lecithin has performed its primary task — that of dissolving cholesterol, fueling creativity, and supporting healthy beautiful skin — it goes on to be used as a high-grade carbohydrate fuel for physical and mental activity. It also supports a general feeling of wellness and positivity and ambition. And lecithin provides an important brain nutrient, choline. A good supply of lecithin can help when a quick reserve of mental energy is needed. Lecithin (choline) rich foods are eggs, soybeans, liver, cauliflower, and cabbage.

Superoxide Dismutase

Superoxide dismutase, or SOD, is the fifth most common protein in the body. It combats and controls chemically reactive free radicals. Since free radicals are damaging to the body's cells, it is necessary to eliminate them. SOD is a powerful antioxidant. Without enzymes such as SOD, humans would quickly die. It helps eliminate the free radicals caused by smoking, and eating dark roasted foods (such as barbecued foods, and roasted beverages such as coffee). It also helps prevent free radical damage from radiation therapy.

The life spans of several mammal species, including man, have been shown to be directly related to their levels of SOD protection. SOD is a naturally occurring zinc and copper containing enzyme that many believe to be linked directly to natural longevity. Richard Cutter, gerontologist, found a proportional relationship between life span and levels of SOD. Studies by Dr. Joseph McCord suggest that SOD can prevent damage to the synovial fluid and membranes caused by arthritis, a common degenerative disease of aging. And SOD has a reputation in the health field as being useful for arthritis relief.

Orgotein, a type of SOD, has been used in Europe since 1981 to reduce inflammation in patients suffering from osteoarthritis and rheumatoid arthritis. Interestingly, it is made in California by an American company, and exported to Europe.

Some people, including some doctors, mistakenly believe that SOD cannot survive the stomach acids. They conclude that none of it gets digested, and therefore is of no value and a waste of money. What they most likely don't know is that the SOD used in original medical research was an unstable SOD isolated from horse blood and beef liver. It had to be injected directly into the bloodstream to get the desired results.

The life spans of several mammal species, including man, have been shown to be directly related to their levels of SOD protection.

Dr. Peter Rothschild, M.D., Ph.D., biochemist, has found in his research that SOD, taken orally, survives in significance all the way to the bloodstream — one hour after consumption. In fact, peroxidase P4D1, an antioxidant enzyme relative of SOD, actually becomes more biologically active when exposed to

Fountain of Youth Secret No. 22

SOD supplementation has been used in Europe to treat arthritis for the past 25 years.

stomach acid. It's almost as if it waits for the stomach acid to hit it so it can jump into action.

Dr. Yoshihide Hagiwara, M.D. says "These enzymes are absorbed directly through membranes in the mouth, throat and stomach... and are more effective when sipped rather than gulped down."

Vegetable sources of SOD, (spirulina, wheat and barley grass, and sprouting seeds) have produced wonderful results and benefits when taken orally. The other nutrients and enzymes in the vegetable sources also work synergistically with your body to help it produce more SOD internally. Dr. Mary Ruth Swope states "Dried barley juice is an excellent natural source of SOD." [15]

Zinc, one of the most important constituents of SOD, is required for growth and healing, and also acts as an antioxidant to help prevent damage to cellular structures. (And many people report anti-cold and anti-viral benefits from additional intake of zinc.)

Liver production of SOD declines from about 1,700 units per gram of body weight at birth to less than 50 units per gram at age eighty. Humans must supplement with SOD as they grow older if they desire the powerful antioxidant and other benefits of this important nutrient.

Footnotes

1. Gale Maleskey, "A Doctor's Guide to Anti-Aging Nutrients", *Prevention*, (Pennsylvania, Rodale Press), 1985

2. From the American Cancer Society, National Research Council, and the National Cancer Institute

3. *Diet, Nutrition and Cancer*, (Washington, National Academy Press), 1982

4. Dr. Arthur Winter, *Bottom Line Personal*, (New York, Boardroom Reports), 1992

5. Maleskey, Prevention, 1985

6. Maleskey, Prevention, 1985

7. A. Hoffer, (New England Journal of Medicine), 1971

8. F. R. Klenner, (Journal of International Academy of Preventative Medicine), 1974 and (Journal of Applied Nutrition), 1971

9. "Bypass Heart Damage with Vitamin E", *Prevention*, (Pennsylvania, Rodale Press), 1987

10. "The Healing Frontier of Vitamin E", *Prevention*, (Pennsylvania, Rodale Press), 1989

11. Med. Welt, 30:411-416, 1979

12. From a paper by P. Fassati and M. Fassati of Carolus University in Prague, at the 1977 symposium held by the Department of Approval of New Drugs and Medico-Technical Aids of the Ministry of Health, U.S.S.R.

13. From a paper presented by M. Marsel Mesulam, M.D., and Sandra Weintraub, Ph.D., of Beth Israel Hospital, Boston, at the International Study Group on Memory Disorders, Zurich, 1979

14. American Journal of Digestive Diseases, 1952

15. Dr. Mary Ruth Swope, *Green Leaves of Barley*

Chapter 7

Minerals and Anti-Aging

People from the beginning of time have recognized the value of minerals. Many remedies and treatments used minerals to relieve various conditions. The Chinese used seaweed for goiter, the Greeks used iron-enriched water to treat anemia, and the people of biblical times used salt as a purifying agent. It was not until the 19th century, however, that research and study of minerals began in a significant fashion. By the early 20th century, minerals, along with vitamins, had been recognized for their importance in human nutrition.

Minerals are actually inorganic substances found in the soil. Plants are able to convert these inorganic minerals into organic ones. Humans eat the plants, and ingest second stage organic minerals. There are those in the health field who believe that humans cannot assimilate inorganic minerals — they must be organic before they become bio-available to our bodies. For this reason, they advocate drinking distilled water, as the body cannot use the inorganic dissolved minerals in spring or well water.

Minerals function as structural components of the body. They also serve as catalysts that regulate other bodily functions.

Importance of Minerals

Minerals function as structural components of the body. They also serve as catalysts that regulate other bodily functions. In this function, they are similar to enzymes in the body. It's been said for years that calcium makes strong bones and teeth, while iron is needed for rich, red blood.

A balanced mineral supplement or food source is probably best for assimilation by the body.

Some experts make a distinction between chelated and non-chelated mineral supplements. Chelated minerals have been produced in such a way that they are bound with a protein molecule. This is done in order to increase the bio-availability of the mineral in the bloodstream. Non-chelated minerals are minerals in their organic state without added proteins. Generally, if there is concern about mineral absorption, the chelated form should be used. They are more expensive to purchase, however. It is the opinion of some that minerals, when taken with meals, do not need to be chelated. And since most supplements are taken with meals, this is not a big concern to most people.

Since many minerals need supplies of other minerals to be effective, one should only use a balanced mineral supplement. Some minerals, such as potassium, are generally not recommended for single-source supplementation. It's better to stay with a multi-mineral supplement, or concentrate on food sources.

Calcium

The Recommended Daily Allowance (RDA) for calcium is 800 mgs., with an upper limit of 1500 mgs. For pregnant or lactating women the figure goes up to 1200 mgs. The 800 mg. requirement equals about three glasses of whole or skim milk daily. It has been estimated that 20% of white adults and 80%

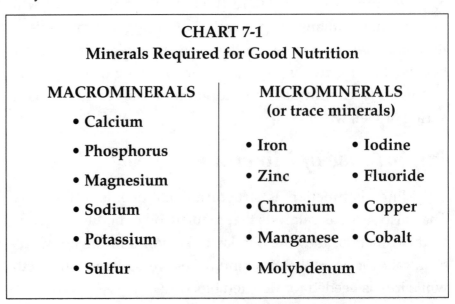

CHART 7-1
Minerals Required for Good Nutrition

MACROMINERALS	MICROMINERALS (or trace minerals)	
• Calcium		
• Phosphorus	• Iron	• Iodine
• Magnesium	• Zinc	• Fluoride
• Sodium	• Chromium	• Copper
• Potassium	• Manganese	• Cobalt
• Sulfur	• Molybdenum	

of black adults cannot digest the lactose present in milk, so supplementation may be needed for those who are lactose intolerant. [1]

People who are lactose intolerant should not use a calcium lactate supplement to meet their calcium needs. Another form of calcium is indicated in that situation.

Of all the calcium in the body, 99% of it is found in the bones and teeth. Since bones are constantly being rebuilt, about 20% of bone calcium is being reabsorbed and replaced each year. [2] Thus the need for regular calcium intake is clear. It is vital in the formation of strong bones and teeth. Of the remaining 1% of calcium not used for the bones or teeth, it is needed for proper muscle function, transmission of nerve impulses, blood clot formation, proper functioning of the parathyroid hormone, structuring of cell membranes, and absorption of vitamin B12. [3]

Although milk and milk products form a large part of the American diet, a USDA survey released in 1969 pointed out that over 30% of the population is calcium deficient. [4]

Inability to digest lactose accounts for part of this, but the aging process is another factor causing this deficiency. With age, the body loses its ability to absorb calcium, leading to softening of the bones (osteoporosis or osteomalacia). In fact, Professor Leo Lutwak of the University of California Medical School has said, "Various surveys have indicated that approximately 30% of women over age 55 and 30% of men over age 60 have sufficient mineral loss to have produced at least one fracture." [5]

In all age groups, calcium deficiency has been associated with impaired muscle function, increased irritability, and poor blood clot formation. The need for calcium seems to be increased by excitement, depression, and excessive bed rest, as well as by the aging process.

A chelate that releases the mineral in ionic form at the intestinal wall, or will be readily absorbed as the intact chelate, will enhance the absorption of that mineral element. It will do so by preventing that mineral from being converted to an

In all age groups, calcium deficiency has been associated with impaired muscle function, increased irritability, and poor blood clot formation.

insoluble chemical compound by preventing its strong absorption on insoluble colloids. [6] Amino acids, acting as chelates, are present normally in meat and poultry proteins. This is why it's recommended taking a mineral supplement with meals. That way, the greatest natural chelation and assimilation is realized.

There are several reasons besides chelation to explain why the calcium in food may not be available to the body: the digestive juices of the stomach may not be acid enough to dissolve insoluble minerals in the food; oxalic acid (in vegetables) or phytic acid (in cereals) can tie up calcium by forming compounds the body cannot absorb; and other foods may render the mineral unusable.

Because amino acid chelates naturally play such an important role in the body, as well as for other reasons, M.L. Scott, Professor of Animal Nutrition at Cornell University wrote "The role of amino acids... in the formation of chelates...should lead to improved diets for the better health of animals, including man." [7]

As the body grows older, it loses its ability to absorb calcium, leading to osteoporosis.

CHART 7-2
Causes of Bone Loss

1. Calcium malabsorption

2. Calcium deficiency

3. Deficiency in estrogen after menopause

4. Availability of vitamin D in the blood

5. Vitamin D utilization in vivo

6. Availability and absorption of vitamin C, magnesium, phosphorous, and fluoride

7. Physical activity level of the individual

8. Increasing age of our population

9. Lactose intolerance or the inability to metabolize milk-sugar complexes

---

Good food sources of calcium include dairy foods, seafood, dark green leafy vegetables, almonds, asparagus, broccoli, cabbage, collards and dandelion greens, figs, kale, kelp, oats, tofu, and whey.

Osteoporosis

Osteoporosis represents a conflict between the normally balanced processes of bone formation and bone loss. If bone is lost through a process called resorption, the mineral content (mostly calcium) is returned to the blood. Over a period of years, osteoporosis can occur if more bone is lost than formed. This may lead to hip, vertebrae, leg or arm bone weakness, resulting in increased trauma and fractures. Therefore, this process leads to the bone failing to perform its supportive function.

Calcium phosphate is the major constituent of bone. Research has shown that dietary calcium requirements may increase with age. Women begin to lose bone during menopause at accelerating rates for 15-20 years and may lose 1/2 to 1-1/2% of their peak bone mass every year. Men also lose bone mass but at a much lower rate. There is no doubt that many people do not have adequate calcium blood levels to replace lost bone.

Both men and women lose bone mass after age 45. Much of that is lost forever due to low calcium levels.

CHART 7-3

Supplemental Calcium Needs

1. Most women over 45 years old (post-menopausal).

2. Some men over 45 years of age.

3. Men and women with smaller, lighter bones in the high risk group.

4. Meat eaters as opposed to vegetarians.

5. Men and women who are older and sedentary.

6. Men and women who cannot absorb calcium.

Two researchers, Forrest Nielsen and Curtiss Hunt, at the Agriculture Department Research Center in Beltsville, Maryland believe they have found why some people with low calcium blood levels also have a low incidence of osteoporosis.

Fountain of Youth Secret No. 23
Calcium supplementation is needed to prevent osteoporosis — especially after age 45.

It's a substance called boron. The blood of women getting boron supplements contained 50% more of a form of estrogen that slows the progression of osteoporosis. They caution that large doses of boron can be dangerous — try eating boron rich foods such as leafy vegetables, nuts, apples, pears, and grapes.

Studies have indicated that older persons absorb calcium at a slower rate than younger persons, but need more to maintain a positive calcium balance. In fact, it is not necessarily the amount of calcium that is significant, but a person's ability to absorb and utilize the calcium that is ingested. [8]

Chromium

The National Research Council suggests daily doses of chromium between 50-200 micrograms. This same daily dose is also recommended by the Food and Nutrition Board of the National Academy of Sciences. Male athletes weighing over 200 pounds can take from 400-600 mcgs. per day.

Chromium and magnesium have been used to help heart disease. Chromium in particular has been shown to protect against heart disease and high blood pressure. A number of studies done as far back as ten years ago showed that the nations with the lowest levels of chromium in the adult population had the highest amounts of cardiovascular disease. These same nations also had the highest levels of refined carbohydrate (sugar) intake.

When autopsies were done on individuals who died of heart attacks, biopsies of their major blood vessels failed to show any chromium. Several researchers have found that chromium supplementation lowered not only blood sugar levels but cholesterol as well.

Chromium and magnesium have been used to help heart disease, high blood pressure, and lower cholesterol levels.

The average American diet is chromium-poor. Optimal amounts of biologically active chromium are essential for good health. Some researchers estimate that 2/3 of the American population have some form of blood sugar condition, either diabetic, hypoglycemic, or prehypoglycemic. The inability to regulate blood sugar levels is caused in part by a chromium deficiency.

Chromium ensures that the insulin hormone works efficiently. Insulin is the body's primary anabolic hormone. Without at least minimal amounts of chromium, insulin doesn't work at all. Insulin's primary functions are to regulate the

Fountain of Youth Secret No. 24
Chromium Picolinate has been shown to reduce body fat and increase muscle mass.

metabolism of blood sugars, lipids, and protein. Insulin is also involved in resisting disease by stimulating the immune system. Biologically active chromium is readily assimilable and assists insulin in all of its major functions. Chromium picolinate improves glucose tolerance, can lower cholesterol, and enhance muscle synthesis.

Since it is used to metabolize sugar, chromium is needed for energy. And in this regard, it has been useful in the treatment and prevention of diabetes.

Chromium helps insulin metabolize sugar to produce energy in the body.

Insulin and chromium escort glucose and fat out of the blood and into the cells. They do the same with amino acids. By increasing the flux of aminos into the cells, thereby directing the synthesis of new protein and inhibiting the break-down of protein, insulin can increase muscle mass. Once inside the cells, amino acids are reassembled into protein for hormones, enzymes, organ tissue, and muscle tissue. If biologically active chromium is in short supply, this process becomes inefficient. When biologically active chromium is restored to optimal levels, cellular uptake of amino acid is improved and muscle synthesis is enhanced.

Chromium picolinate, a specific form of chromium, is the most widely studied form of chromium. It is a convertible substance, similar to beta carotene, in that it converts into elemental chromium at a 12.7% rate. Therefore, the daily dose for chromium picolinate can be from 394-1574 mcgs., and from 3150-4724 mcgs. for athletes. This picolinate form has received much attention for its use in body fat reduction and muscle mass increase.

Food sources for chromium include brown rice, cheese, meat, whole grains, dried beans, chicken, corn, calves' liver, mushrooms, and potatoes. Of interest is that no side effects have been found to date from chromium supplementation.

Iron

Iron deficient anemia has been recorded as early as 1500 B.C. in Egypt. That's why iron has earned its well deserved reputation as a blood builder. In fact, the single most important function of this mineral is its production of hemoglobin, and supplying red blood cells with oxygen. This is also the mineral found in the largest amounts in the blood.

Iron is important for growth in children and resistance to disease. It's required for a healthy immune system, and for the proper regulation of neurotransmitters in the brain.

Iron is involved in the entire breathing process. Cytochromes and cytochrome oxidase are proteins and enzymes necessary for cell metabolism and cell respiration. They simply do not work without iron. Iron is also important for collagen and elastin production. These are the two major components of connective tissues in the body.

The RDA varies with age — adult men can take up to 10 mg. daily. Women can take up to 18 mg. daily (reducing that to 10 mg. daily after age 50). Pregnant women need 30-60 mg. a day. Lactating women need 30-60 mg. per day up to three months after delivery, reducing after that to 18 mg. per day.

Food sources include eggs, fish, liver, meat, poultry, dark green leafy vegetables, whole grains, beets, almonds, dates, kelp, kidney, lentils, kidney and lima beans, rice and wheat bran, and soybeans.

Magnesium

The National Research Council recommends 350 mg. of magnesium a day for men and 300 mg. daily for women.

Iron is needed for proper respiratory processes and cellular metabolism.

Fountain of Youth Secret No. 25
Magnesium supplementation is essential for anyone eating the typical American diet.

Dietary intake may be inadequate in large segments of the population. The average American diet contains about 120 mgs. of magnesium. Magnesium is vital to enzyme activity. It is quite clearly required for human life. It protects the arterial linings from stress, and helps prevent muscle weakness, heart disease, high blood pressure, and aids in maintaining the proper ph balance.

It is also needed for the electrical functions of the cells, muscle contraction, and heart strength.

Magnesium deficiency is becoming more prevalent. Especially at risk are the elderly, diabetics, regular consumers of alcohol, pregnant women, and people who exercise strenuously.

Food sources include dairy products, fish, meat, seafood, apples, bananas, brown rice, garlic, kelp, lima beans, nuts, peaches, tofu, green leafy vegetables, and whole grains.

Potassium

The suggested daily intake of potassium is between 1875 - 5625 mgs. per day.

Potassium is needed for a good nervous system, and regular heart rhythms. It helps prevent stroke, aids in muscle use, and synergizes with sodium to regulate the body's fluid balance.

Food sources include dairy foods, fish, fruit, meat, poultry, vegetables, and whole grains.

Footnotes

1. C.C. Pfeiffer, " Mental and Elemental Nutrients", *A Physicians Guide to Nutrition and Health Care* (New Canaan, CT: Keats Publishing,1975)

2. E.D. Wilson, K.H. Fisher, and M.E. Fuqua, *Principles of Nutrition, 3rd ed.*, (New York, John Wiley & Sons), 1975

3. Pfeiffer, and Wilson, et al.

4. Pfeiffer

5. L. Lutwak, *Geriatrics*, 1974

6. J.J. Mortvedt, P.M. Giordano, W.W. Lindsay, eds., "Micronutrients in Agriculture", *Soil Science Society of America* (Madison, WI)

7. M.L. Scott in Mortvedt, et al.

8. Patricia Ireland and John Fordtran, "Effect of Dietary Calcium and Age on Jejunal Calcium Absorption in Humans Studies by Intestinal Perfusion," *The Journal of Clinical Investigation*, Nov. 1983, Vol. 52, and Ron L. Miller, M.D., "Accelerated Bone Loss in an Aged Woman," *Journal of the American Geriatrics Society*, June, 1984, Vol. 32, No. 6

Chapter 8

Coenzyme Q10 and Anti-Aging

As already discussed, enzymes are protein substances found in plants, animals, humans, and all living things. They are necessary for the building and rebuilding of cells and tissues, and are made up of at least two parts: the protein portion and the cofactor portion. Mineral ions or vitamins make up the cofactor portion of the complete enzyme; the vitamin portion is usually called the coenzyme.

The body uses food to obtain the enzymes Q1 through Q10. The liver then manufactures coenzyme Q10 from all these components. Coenzyme Q10 is the only Q enzyme that the body uses at the cellular level.

Quite plainly, coenzyme Q10 is the most exciting nutritional discovery in the last thirty years.

Every cell in the body needs Q10 for energy and proper metabolism

Q10 and the Energy Cycle

As was mentioned in Chapter One, coenzyme Q10 is an essential component of the mitochondrial energy cycle. It plays a critical role in our entire energy process. The mitochondria use this enzyme and ADP to create all cellular energy. Since the ATP supply is limited to only about 3 ounces in the entire body at any given time, an ongoing conversion process must take place. For this conversion, Q10 is necessary. Without adequate levels of Q10, the mitochondria cannot supply the cells with enough ATP for energy conversion. So as a result the body becomes susceptible to a wide range of conditions of ill health.

FIGURE 8-1
ThePower of Co-Enzyme Q10

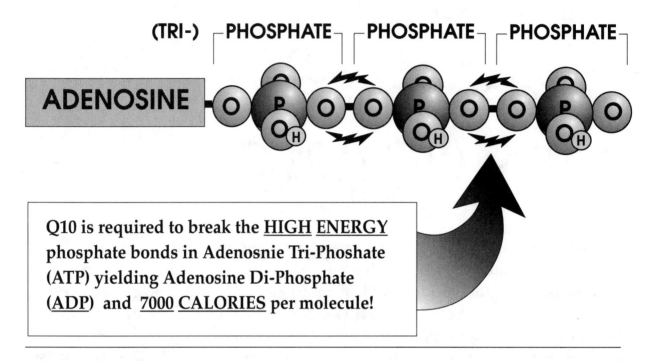

Q10 is required to break the <u>HIGH</u> <u>ENERGY</u> phosphate bonds in Adenosnie Tri-Phoshate (ATP) yielding Adenosine Di-Phosphate (<u>ADP</u>) and <u>7000</u> <u>CALORIES</u> per molecule!

The Relationship Between Coenzyme Q10 Deficiencies and the Aging Process

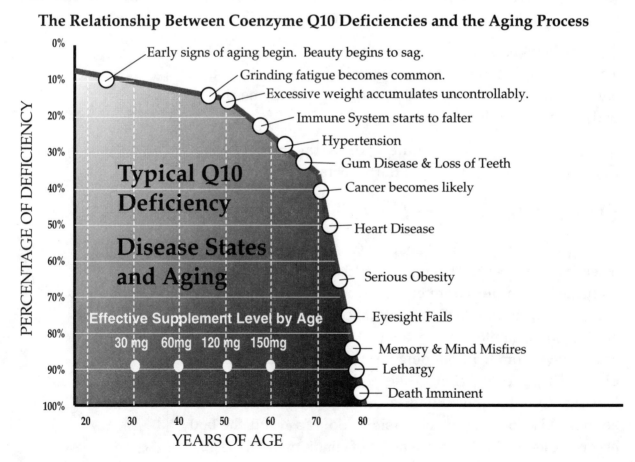

Coenzyme Q10 is found in every cell of the body. Sometimes called ubiquinone, coenzyme Q10 is a naturally occurring substance similar in molecular structure to some vitamins. The body must have energy available to perform even the simplest operation — that's why Q10 is considered essential for the body's cells. Q10 is the only Q enzyme used in the human body. It produces energy, is a catalyst for bodily reactions, and is also a powerful antioxidant.

Studies from around the world confirm Q10's anti-aging benefits.

Results of Research Studies

Discovered in the early 1960's by Dr. F.L. Crane at the University of Wisconsin, Q10 originally cost over $450,000.00 dollars a pound. Since then, scientists have discovered how to isolate and grow it economically. Now it can be purchased at reasonable prices in various milligram doses.

Hundreds of studies from Japan, the Soviet Union, Europe, and the U.S. have shown coenzyme Q10 to be literally miraculous in its ability to normalize the function of each of the body's 69 trillion cells and helps to dramatically roll back the aging process and the effects of time. Coenzyme Q10 helps bring about all of the following: increased energy, courage, ambition, radiant beauty, real weight loss, mental power, vibrant sexuality, a feeling of well-being, a positive nature, a vigorous healing and immune system, and a healthy heart and circulatory system. It truly is a fountain of life and energy.

Q10 Production Levels and Age

Q10 increases energy, improves heart function, and provides radiant beauty, natural weight control and vibrant sexuality.

As the body ages, the liver's production of coenzyme Q10 declines. That is why everyone needs to supplement with Q10. One study found that Q10 declines by up to 80% in the course of normal aging. Deficiencies approaching 80% have been found in elderly people with serious heart disease.

Coenzyme Q10 levels begin to decline in the body about the age of 17-18 years old. Before that, it remains relatively high. This explains why energy levels drop when a person reaches their early 20's. By age 30, the body is about 11% deficient, and by age 40, about 14% deficient. This is the period when fatigue becomes common, and excess weight adds on almost uncontrollably.

Deficiency levels above 30% increase the likelihood of cancer, obesity, heart disease, lethargy, failing eyesight, and mind and memory problems. To return coenzyme Q10 levels to childhood levels, with a corresponding increase in energy, supplementation with 10-30 mg. per day or higher is needed. In demanding situations, one can supplement with as much as 120 milligrams.

Coenzyme Q10 oral supplementation results in increased energy levels, improvement of heart function, prevention and cure of gum disease, and possible life extension. It is critical for energy, ambition, radiant beauty, weight control, mental power, and vibrant sexuality. Q10 is absolutely the most important enzyme for the body's energy levels.

Q10 Helps Heart Problems

The greatest amount of coenzyme Q10 is found in the heart and liver, which accounts for its positive results in the treatment of cardiovascular disease, angina pectoris, congestive heart failure, cardiomyopathy, hyperthyroid heart failure, mitral valve prolapse, and hypertension.

Biopsies done on the heart tissue of individuals with a variety of heart problems have shown that 50-75% of them have been deficient in Q10. Studies have clearly shown the beneficial effect of Q10 supplementation on angina pectoris, congestive heart failure, cardiomyopathy, mitral valve prolapse, high blood pressure, and heart toxicity from a variety of medical drugs.

In angina patients, it decreased their episodes of angina by as much as 53%, and significantly increased their ability to do the treadmill test. These individuals were given 150 mgs. daily for four weeks. In numerous studies of congestive heart failure patients, over 50% of the participants were consistently helped by Q10 doses of approximately 30 mgs. daily. In the cardiomyopathies, 100 mg. daily of Q10 gave improvements to 82% of the patients. In high blood pressure individuals, 60 mgs. daily resulted in a 10% reduction of blood pressure in over 91% of those treated.

Doctors Use Q10 with Heart Patients

Coenzyme Q10 has been used by doctors to treat heart failure at the Methodist Hospital in Indianapolis and the Institute for Biomedical Research at the University of Texas. Doctors and researchers found that 91% of their heart patients showed improvement within thirty days of beginning coenzyme Q10 supplementation.

The American Journal of Cardiology printed research on coenzyme Q10's effects in relieving the painful heart condition angina pectoris. Research at the Free University in Brussels demonstrated that Q10 boosts the performance of the heart, even with severe cardiac disease. Research at the University of Texas found a three year 75% survival rate for congestive heart failure patients, compared to a 25% survival rate for conventional medical treatment. And they also found, along with the Center for Adult Diseases in Japan, that Q10 lowers high blood pressure.

Q10 boosts survival rate of severe cardiac patients by 300% and lowers high blood pressure.

Q10 Aids Life Extension

In laboratory animal studies, Coenzyme Q10 extended life-span by up to 56%. If all this holds true in humans, man could expect to live to over 100 years of age, and do it with energy and vitality.

A number of studies on animals have proven the immune-enhancing effect of Coenzyme Q10. Several studies have shown that the germ-killing ability of white blood cells

---

CHART 8-1
Cardiovascular Benefits of Coenzyme Q10

- Reduces congestive heart failure by strengthening the heart muscle.

- Reduces cardiac arrhythmias and chance of heart attack.

- Lowers blood pressure.

- Reduces injury from stroke or heart attack.

increased after Q10 was given. Other germ-killing cells also increased in number after supplementation. Q10 also prolonged the lives of animals after they had been infected with a number of pathogenic organisms.

A Q10 deficiency could cause or aggravate many medical conditions, thereby lessening life expectancy.

In older animals, immune system deficiency was partially reversed with Q10 supplementation. It may be possible that using it on a regular basis will help to reverse age-related immune system decline.

In human studies of patients with various diseases, (diabetes, cancer, and heart problems) significant increases in the level of immunoglobulin G were found in the patient's serum. This increase could represent a boosting of the immune system.

According to studies done by Dr. Karl Folkers, director of the Institute for Biomedical Research at the University of Texas, once coenzyme Q10 levels drop below 25% of normal, disease

---

CHART 8-2
Anti-Aging Benefits of Coenzyme Q10

- Increases energy.

- Increases exercise tolerance.

- Helps correct age related decline in the immune system.

- Defuses harmful peroxides (free radicals) within the body.

- Stimulates the immune system.

- Protects mitochondrial membranes with its powerful antioxidant properties.

- Provides honest weight loss.

- Increases mental power.

- Promotes vibrant sexuality.

- Creates a feeling of well-being and a positive nature.

may develop. And if levels drop below 75%, death may follow as a natural consequence.

Deficiencies of coenzyme Q10 have been reported in a range of clinical conditions. Supplementation guards against deficiency, and is considered safe and effective. Poor eating

---

Fountain of Youth Secret No. 26
Adequate levels of Coenzyme Q10 are required for a healthy heart, long life, and abundant energy.

---

habits, stress, and infection adversely affect the body's ability to produce adequate amounts of Q10. Necessary for energy production, a deficiency could cause or aggravate many medical conditions, thereby lessening life expectancy.

In patients with periodontal disease, it was found that their gum tissues demonstrated deficiencies of coenzyme Q10. Patients with advanced periodontal disease who received supplemental Q10 healed 2-3 times faster than usual following surgery.

Q10 and Diabetes

Diabetes is a disorder of carbohydrate metabolism. It is the result of insufficient production or utilization of insulin in the bloodstream. In most instances, it is a result of genetics and heredity, but it may also result from a deficiency of beta cells. This can be caused by inflammation, surgery, or other unknown problems. As discussed in Chapter Seven, chromium plays a role in the process of metabolizing carbohydrates and empowering insulin.

Animal studies have shown that diabetic animals are deficient in the Q10 enzyme.

Q10 is also involved in carbohydrate metabolism. Animal studies have shown that diabetic animals are deficient in the enzyme. Supplementation of Q10 partially corrected the abnormal glucose metabolism problems.

A daily dose of 120 mgs. caused fasting blood sugar to drop up to 30% in 26 of the 39 people tested, for a success rate of 66%.

At this time, the exact process that Q10 uses to correct or improve diabetic control is not known. Two views have been offered: one is that Q10 helps the body synthesize more of the Q10 enzyme itself. The second view is that somehow Q10 helps to improve carbohydrate metabolism. Certainly, more work is needed in this clinical condition. Regardless of how it works, supplementation today can be done easily and safely to reap the many benefits of this wonder enzyme.

Q10 and Excess Weight

As discussed in Chapter 2, when a person takes in more calories than they burn, they gain weight. There are any number of ways to correct this imbalance: reduce calorie intake, exercise more, or increase the body's heat output through a process called thermogenics.

It is known that some people do not produce as much heat energy as others. In some cases, an overweight condition can be caused by inadequate metabolic activity. One easy way to check for this situation is to determine body temperature immediately upon awakening. Do this by placing an oral thermometer under the arm for 10 minutes. After checking for 5-10 days, if the average awakening temperature is 97.6° fahrenheit or lower, this may indicate a slow metabolism. Thermogenic herbal formulas are available to counteract slow metabolism. It may also be appropriate to review this situation with a health care provider.

In 1984, 27 very obese individuals were tested for Q10 levels. Over 50% were found to be deficient in Q10. Two groups were tested; the first group was deficient in Q10, the second group was not. After nine weeks of 100 mgs. of Q10 daily, the first group had lost an average of 29 pounds, while the second group lost only an average of 12 pounds.

A daily Q10 dose of 120 mg. caused fasting blood sugar to drop up to 30% in 26 of the 39 people tested — success rate of 66%.

While this is only one study, it indicates that some overweight individuals may be up to 50% deficient in Q10. Perhaps this is one reason why many people have little if any success with most diet plans — a Q10 deficiency may play a large part in their excess weight.

Therefore, combining a reduced calorie diet with Q10 supplementation may result in satisfactory weight loss when other methods have failed.

Q10 Used by Millions for Years

Q10 has been used for many years in Japan. Over 15 million Japanese people use it every month — could this be the reason for their reputation of having abundant energy? Since 1974, it has been used by the Japanese as a cardiac medicine. Americans are just finding out about this wonderful nutrient.

After nine weeks of daily dose of 100 mgs. of Q10, a Q10 deficient group lost an average of 29 pounds, the non-deficient group lost an average of 12 pounds.

CHART 8-3
Additional Medical Benefits of Coenzyme Q10

• Fighting periodontal disease

• Counteracting damage from some drug therapy

• Enhances the pumping ability of the heart and circulatory system.

• Prevents and helps cure gum disease

• Helps cardiovascular disease:
  Angina pectoris
  Congestive heart failure
  Cardiomyopathy
  Hyperthyroid heart failure
  Mitral valve prolapse
  Hypertension

• Vigorously helps the healing and immune system

• Provides honest weight loss

Coenzyme Q10 has been used by millions on a daily basis in doses of 10-30mg. Therapeutic doses of 100 mgs. or more have been used. No serious adverse effects of any kind have been reported with long-term use. Q10 should not be used during pregnancy or lactation simply because it has not yet been proven for use during these periods.

It may take up to three months to saturate deficient tissues, because the synthesis of new coenzyme Q10 dependent enzymes is a slow process.

Using a green superfood, you can get the Q10 equivalent of 130 pounds of raw broccoli per day. One bottle of coenzyme Q10 supplements roughly equals one ton of raw broccoli. And using Q10 capsules as oral supplements makes getting this vital enzyme to the cells quick and easy.

Rich food sources of Q10 are beef heart, mackerel, sardines, and other meats and fish. Cereals, brans, peanuts, dark leafy green vegetables, and soybeans are good sources as well.

Chapter 9

Swedish Pollen Extract

Pollen as the Perfect Food

The Father of Medicine, Hippocrates, once stated, "Let your food be your medicine and your medicine be your food." Almost since the beginning of time, man has used pollen as a high-quality food. One of man's earliest foods was pollen. Cave drawings show honey hunters harvesting this food. The Bible, Roman writings, and other early narratives refer to the benefits of honey and pollen. Homer referred to it as "the food of kings," and guests in Roman homes were welcomed with the words, "Here is honey and pollen, provided by the gods, to protect your health."

Pollen well deserves its reputation as nature's most perfect food.

In the Orient, honey and pollen were used as a supplement to the diet. It is even believed by some that John the Baptist in the Bible ate pollen with honey as a mainstay of his diet. Many people the world over recognize the value of pollen for good health, good eating, and its healthy qualities. Pollen well deserves its reputation as nature's most perfect food.

Researchers have found that a diet including pollen has actually retarded development of tumors in lab mice with cancer. Sociologists and scientists studying populations with advanced old age members have found that a long life of vigor and health can be traced largely to a diet high in fiber and pollen.

Researchers in Sweden, Germany, and Belgium have documented evidence that pollen improves prostate disorders. Professor Alin Caillas, French agriculturist and laureate of the Academy of Agriculture, reports that 35 grams of pollen daily would satisfy most of the nutritional requirements for the average person.

Two Types of Pollen

BEE POLLEN — THE BAD POLLEN

Many centenarians in the world work as beekeepers. In so doing, they keep the dark honey for themselves — it's a far richer source of bee pollen.

They know that queen bees grow three times larger and live ten times longer with incredible fertility compared to the genetically identical worker bees. This occurs because they are fed a pollen extract food called "royal jelly" from the time they are born. The worker bees make royal jelly by taking pollen into their mouths, mixing it with special enzymes from glands in their heads, and expelling the liquid.

Notwithstanding the belief of these beekeepers, bee pollen is actually a bad food. There are a number of reasons for this which need further discussion.

It is impossible to control what bees harvest. They will gather pollen or nectar from almost any source. In fact, they may gather pollen from a plant that causes allergic reactions. To ingest bee pollen that contains allergens will likely cause an adverse response in an allergic individual. It can well be said that bee pollen may actually aggravate allergies.

The quality of bee pollen (actually the lack of quality) is graded by the level of contamination from bee wings, legs, fly eggs, rodent hair and dung, and other foreign matter.

The quality of bee pollen (actually the lack of quality) is graded by the level of contamination from bee wings, legs, fly eggs, rodent hair and dung, and other foreign matter. Allergy symptoms or other harmful physiological responses can occur from these pollutants.

What most people believe is bee pollen is really nectar - the sweet sticky substance on flowers that bees collect to make honey. As much as 96% of what people call bee pollen is really nectar. For many people, the energy that they get from eating "bee pollen" is primarily a sugar lift from this sweet nectar.

Because of this sweet, moist nectar coating on the bee pollen, and the fact that bee pollen is kept in a dark, warm beehive, it becomes a perfect breeding ground for molds and bacteria. Pollen researchers have identified more than 126 varieties of fungus, bacteria, and yeast that grow on the external mucus surface of bee collected pollen. If a person has an allergy to mold, yeast, or bacteria, ingesting bee pollen can be very harmful, and will likely cause an allergy attack.

A very high percentage of people are allergic to the contaminants in bee pollen, especially the high content of bacteria, mold, and fungus in the sweet nectar. For many people, the "rush" felt from taking bee pollen is really an allergic reaction to the contaminants.

An even greater surprise is that bee pollen cannot be digested by the human body. Every pollen grain has an outer covering, like a nut, which cannot be broken down in the human digestive tract. Only about 3% of the pollen food inside this shell is digested out through an opening in the pollen grain called the hila. This means that about 97% of the bee pollen passes through our system undigested. That makes it a real waste of money, and of little if any nutritional value.

It should be re-emphasized that the major problem with bee pollen is not in the pollen itself, but rather the collection and storage methods used by the bee. These poor conditions are of no consequence to the bee, but extremely detrimental to humans. For people concerned about health and nutrition, bee pollen remains a poor food, and for people with allergies, it can be dangerous.

SWEDISH POLLEN EXTRACT — THE GOOD POLLEN

Swedish pollen extract has none of the problems of bee pollen. Harvested without bees by a mechanical harvesting machine, select pollens with ideal micronutrient profiles for humans are extracted with none of the pollutants or contaminants common to bee pollen. Swedish pollen is highly processed and pre-digested with live enzymes to make this

> **Pollen researchers have identified more than 126 varieties of fungus, bacteria, and yeast that grow on the external mucus surface of bee-collected pollen.**

pharmaceutical-grade product hypoallergenic. It contains none of the molds, bacteria, and other contaminants of bee pollen.

Today's pollen extract product is derived from a blend of pollens from select flowers, cereal grasses (superfood-type), and conifers that Swedish scientists have identified as having a broad spectrum of micronutrients. Swedish pollen is a superior food supplement which ensures a balanced supply of vital nutrients in a concentrated form. It supplies vital nutrients to the body and cells, including all essential amino acids, unsaturated fatty acids, enzymes, and numerous carbohydrates, vitamins, minerals, and trace elements. It improves the absorption of vitamins, minerals and trace elements from the food we eat, and releases energy in every cell in the body.

Processed in Sweden by a purely mechanical process, the pollen is purified and mixed with enzymes to break down the outer pollen covering and reduce the molecular weight of the pollen grains. Only pollen manufactured in this way has such great value to our bodies. Swedish pollen is 100% pure food, and is easily digested by the body. It's the most concentrated nutrient-rich whole food in the world. Pollen processed in this manner becomes a high-grade pollen extract, full of vitamins, minerals, enzymes, micronutrients, RNA, DNA, antioxidants, hormones, and other nutrients.

Nutritionally classified as a superfood, some professional nutritionists believe this to be the single most important food a person can eat. Swedish pollen extract itself is far superior to bee pollen or even beehive royal jelly. And the Swedes are very particular about cleanliness and nutrient supplements, especially so in the factory that processes Swedish pollen. Many professional nutritionists believe that it is the highest-quality pollen product in the world.

Pollen and Allergies

Swedish pollen extract prevents or eliminates many of the symptoms of allergies. It has been tested for these benefits in Italy, Switzerland, and Argentina, and has shown a remarkable effect under these controlled clinical conditions.

Swedish pollen supplies vital nutrients to the body and cells, including all essential amino acids, unsaturated fatty acids, enzymes, and numerous carbohydrates, vitamins, minerals, and trace elements.

As already discussed, many airborne pollen allergies are caused by the fungi and bacteria living on the outside of the pollen grain, and not the pollen itself. Swedish pollen is hypoallergenic since it undergoes a unique natural process to break down the molecules which generally cause allergies. It's an established doctrine of science that small and low molecular weight molecules are generally not allergens. Swedish pollen also apparently works on relieving allergy symptoms by correcting whatever imbalance in the body caused the elevated histamine production in the first place. Pollen-allergenic people should still consult their physician before beginning a pollen-supplementation program.

Since it is free of harmful allergens and pesticide chemical residues, even those who are allergic to the molds and bacteria on bee pollen can enjoy the benefits of Swedish pollen. People highly allergic to hayfever allergens have taken Swedish Pollen without any problems. It has reduced their hayfever symptoms to almost nothing. (Some people, previously incapacitated by allergies, now report sneezing once or twice a day as their only symptoms during the heavy hayfever seasons.)

Scientific Information on Pollen

All plant life begins with fertilization by the microscopic pollen grains. It takes about 6 grains to be seen by the human eye. It takes 400 of some of the smaller pollen grains to equal one millimeter in length.

Plants grow, and animals eat them for food. It could well be argued, and quite reasonably, that all life on earth would cease without pollen. Plants would not germinate and grow, and animals and man would have no food to sustain themselves. Without pollen, man and animals would die of starvation. It's required for plants to grow, both for human food and food for animals.

Pollen has more important biofactors than any other substance known to man. Scientists have identified all 22 amino acids, 27 mineral salts, many enzymes and vitamins including A,C,D, and B complex in pollen. Some researchers believe that it contains every substance needed to maintain life.

Scientists have identified all 22 amino acids, 27 mineral salts, many enzymes and vitamins including A,C,D, and B complex in pollen.

The highly complex pollen molecule is the richest full-spectrum source of amino acids, short peptides, nucleic acids (RNA & DNA), vitamins, minerals, trace elements, fatty acids, phytosterols, terpenes, aliphatic alcohols, flavonoids, coenzymes, and prostaglandin precursors found in nature. In

---

Fountain of Youth Secret No. 27
Swedish Pollen Extract provides almost every nutrient necessary for long life, health and vitality.

---

total, pollen contains well over 100 biologically active components.

Many of its components act as catalysts, utilizing food values that would normally be lost. Researchers have reasoned therefore that pollen builds up one's immune system. Due to this, pollen has also been associated with improved digestion, and extending one's normal life span. It has been reported that a large percentage of the oldest people in more remote parts of the world have been beekeepers. Typically, they kept the darkest (pollen-rich) honey at the bottom of the beehive for themselves. While this bee pollen is a vastly inferior product to today's Swedish pollen, it nonetheless provided a small amount of nutritional benefits.

It has been reported that a large percentage of the oldest people in more remote parts of the world have been beekeepers.

As Chapter one details, cell mitochondria create ATP from Q10, ADP, and fats and carbohydrates. When the cell needs energy, it takes ATP and converts it to ADP, releasing energy in the process. Pollen helps the cells release the maximum amount of energy during the ATP cycle. In so doing, the cells get energized and the body feels full of energy.

The pollen shell is very strong. It is indigestible by the human body (unless treated with enzymes) and can last for

CHART 9-1
Chemical Analysis of Pollen Extract

Vitamins:
Provitamin A
  (Carotenoids)
B1 Thiamine
B2 Riboflavin
Niacin
B6 Pyridoxine
Rutin
Biotin
B12
Folic Acid
Choline
Inositol
Vitamin C
Vitamin D
Vitamin E
Vitamin K
Pantothenic Acid

Minerals
Calcium
Phosphorus
Potassium
Sulphur
Sodium
Chlorine
Magnesium
Iron
Manganese
Copper
Iodine
Zinc
Silicon
Chromium
Molybdenum
Boron
Titanium

Carotenoids:

Beta-carotene	Xanthophylls
Zeaxanthin	Lycopene
Crocetin	

Dietary Essential Amino Acids and Physiological Essential Amino Acids:

Dietary Essential:	Physiologically Essential:
Histidine	Alanine
Isoleucine	Alpha-Amino-
Leucine	Butyric-Acid
Lycine	Arginine
Methionine	Asparagine
Phenylalanine	Aspartic Acid
Threonine	Cysteine
Tryptophan	Cystine
Valine	Glutamic Acid
	Glutamine
	Glycine
	Hydroxyproline
	Proline
	Serine
	Tyrosine

Prostaglandins:
A group of hormone-like compounds derived from linoleic and arachidonic acids that influence innumerable body processes.

Phystosterols:

Fucosterol	Campesterol
Beta-sitosterol	Estrone
Stigmasterol	

Enzymes:
24 Oxidoreductases
21 Transferases
32 Hydrolases
10 lyases
5 Isomerases
2 Ligases and Others

Fatty Acid Profile: Number of C-atoms and double bonds

Caprylic (C-6)
Capric (C-10)
Lauric (C-12)
Myristic (C-14)
Myristoleic (C-14) 1 dbl. bond
Pentadecanoic (C-15)
Pentadecenoic (C-15) 1 dbl. bond
Palmitic (C-16)
Palmitoleic (C-) 1 dbl. bond
Heptadecanoic (C-17)
Heptadecenoic (C-17) 1 dbl. bond
Stearic (C-IX)
Oleic (C-13) 1 dbl. bond
Linoleic (C-13) 1 dbl. bond
Linolenic (C-13) 2 dbl. bonds
Arachidic (C-20)
Eicosenoic (C-20) 1 dbl. bond
Eicosadienoic (C-20) 2 dbl. bonds
Eicosadienoic (C-20) 3 dbl. bonds
Arachidonic (C-20) 4 dbl. bonds

Low Molecular Weight Sugars and Related Compounds:

Fructose	Glucose
Mannose	Xylose
Galactose	Xylitol
Arabinose	Xylogalacturonan
Ribose	Glucoronolactone
Fucose	Raffinose
Hexasamine	Stachyose
Rhamnose	Sucrose
Maltotetratose	
Maltose	
Maltotriose	
Callose	

Flavonoids:

Quercetin	Apigenin
Kaempferol	Dihydroxquercertin
Narigenin	Myricetin
Luteolin	Isorhamnetin

Long Chain Hydrocarbons:

n-pentacosane	Myo-inositol
n-heptacosane	Pinitol
n-nonacosane	Sequitol
n-tricosane	

Growth Regulators:

Auxins	Brassins
Gibberellins	Kinins

Different Classes of Lipids in Flower Pollen:

Polar lipids
The major fractions of the polar lipids in flower pollen are lecithin, lysolecithin, phosphoinositol and physphatidylcholine.

Natural lipids
Monoglycerides
Diglycerides
Triglycerides
Free fatty acids
Sterols
Hydrocarbons

Others:

Chlorophyll	Guanine
Nucleic Acids	Amines
Phenolic Acids	Hexodecanal
Vanillie	Gallic
P. coumaric	Ferulic
Protocatechuic	Pentosans
P. hydroxybenzoic	Terpenes
Nucleosides Vernine	
Xanthine Hypoxanthine Nuclein	

Unknown:
Some of the greatest values of Flower Pollen may stem from elements which are for the moment still unknown to science, and from the synergistic action of all the elements working together.

IMPORTANT: There are established Recommended Daily Allowances for many vitamins and minerals and Flower Pollen contains trace amounts of these ingredients. There is no RDA or established need for the majority of ingredients listed in this Chemical Analysis.

The new "pollen-pistil" product contains the highest grade of stable Super Oxide Dismutase (SOD) in the entire plant world.

thousands of years. Occasionally a story will print in the press about seeds or pollen granules being found at an archaeological digging that are still biologically active. Some seeds found in the Egyptian pyramids have been planted in the ground and still germinated and grew after all these centuries.

Once sold to Americans in a chemically extracted form, Swedish pollen is now available in a non-chemical extraction product. Dr. B. P. Poovaiah, the world's foremost authority on Swedish pollen extract, spearheaded this effort. This new formulation represents an important scientific advance in pollen research for a more pure, potent, and perfect pollen extract. There are no chemical residues in this newly extracted pollen.

Until 1973, pollen extract was made using the same procedures developed back in the early 1950's when pollen extract was first discovered. In 1973, a new pollen product was developed using non-chemical extraction and enzymatic pre-digestion for an astoundingly different and superior pollen extract product. These new pollen products have seen widespread use and success in Europe.

Without question, the culmination of forty years of pollen research is the miracle of the new "pollen-pistil" product. This Swedish pollen product consists of hand-harvested female pistils combined with corresponding male pollens in a special chamber. The combining of these two plant substances creates the greatest release of energy in the plant kingdom. This transforms the pollen into a much higher bio-available form with the highest grade of stable superoxide dismutase (SOD) in the entire plant world. SOD is nature's best antioxidant for rejuvenating cells and tissues in the body. As discussed earlier, SOD is an important anti-aging free radical scavenger that helps rid the body of those dangerous electrons. (See Chapter Five for a complete discussion on SOD.)

Pollen and Sex

Pollen, as the male cell of the plant kingdom, has a well-deserved reputation for extra vim, vigor, and virility. It provides all the biofactors that are precursors for the sex hormones, and micro-nutrients essential for healthy reproductive systems. Exclusive animal breeders in Europe pay top dollar for pollen concentrates that are added to their animals' food. Likewise, some couples report that pollen supplementation enabled them to have children. Many couples also report increased sex drive and increased fertility.

Today, pollen extract is a remedy used by European and Japanese doctors for prostatitis, urethritis, and other conditions of the reproductive organs.

At about 45 years of age, most men experience an enlargement of the prostate gland. This has various symptoms, most notably that of restricting urine flow and poor emptying of the bladder. Other more irritating symptoms usually occur also, such as pain while urinating, frequent nighttime trips to the bathroom, hesitancy, and loss of bladder control.

The most widely used treatment today is a surgical process called prostatectomy. About 350,000 of these procedures are done every year in America. This surgery requires a hospital stay of several days, and a substantial recovery time.

Since the prostate is a secondary sex gland, hormonal drugs have been used to shrink and reduce inflammation. Hormonal inhibitors and neurological blockers are commonly prescribed. These drugs have unpleasant and undesirable side effects, especially in elderly patients.

Interestingly, prostate trouble is unknown in castrated males. Until the late 19th century, castration was a popular treatment for prostate enlargement. For obvious reasons, that treatment has not proved to be very popular.

In Europe, many herbs and plants, under license to pharmaceutical-quality manufacturers, have been used to treat patients with prostate enlargement. Swedish pollen extracts have been used to treat prostate disease for over twenty years.

Recent pharmacological studies and controlled, double-blind clinical trials performed at well-known university centers in England, Germany, Japan, Switzerland and Sweden show that pollen extracts have a significant effect on prostate enlargement by reducing inflammation. In fact, these studies

Recent pharmacological studies and clinical trials show that pollen extracts have a significant effect on prostate enlargement by reducing inflammation.

show that pollen extracts are as effective as all forms of pharmacological medication. Taken daily, pollen provides symptomatic relief from frequent urinations and reduces the amount of urine retained in the bladder.

In a report published in 1985 in Pharmacometrics, volume 31, number 1, Professor Ito confirmed that pollen extract significantly inhibited the increase in prostate weight. Chemical testing showed that the reduced weight of the prostate gland did not hinder its function. In this test, the direct specificity of pollen extract and the prostate was confirmed. Toxicity was very low, and pollen extract positively affected the prostate hypertrophy with very little side effect.

Another report confirmed that the active ingredients in pollen extract stimulate the bladder muscles and act on the urinary tube and outlet to support the flow of urine.

In Europe, pollen formulas have been used for almost forty years. Pharmacies and grocery stores routinely stock Swedish pollen as an over-the-counter nutrient, especially for prostate problems. Pollen is used throughout the world to treat prostatitis and prostate trouble.

Pollen and Athletics

Pollen's greatest reputation is probably on the field of athletic and physical performance. Many world class athletes from various countries have increased their endurance and strength with pollen. Dedicated weight lifters, runners, and body builders are discovering that pollen is a natural and safe alternative to the very dangerous steroid drugs, with none of the side effects. Pollen is completely natural, and works with the body's physiology.

Pollen is widely used by European athletes, and the Finnish and Swedish national Olympic teams. They report that it increases training capacity, strength and stamina, accelerates transportation of nutrients to the cells, fights fatigue, and expands anaerobic ability.

Finnish athletes, in an attempt to supplement their diet, began taking pollen in the 1969 training season. These athletes

It is rumored that Olympic coach Bella Karolyi gave pollen to his world-class gymnasts, including Nadia Comanech, Olga Korbut, Julie McNamara, and Mary Lou Retton.

needed about 5000 calories per day, as well as ample amounts of protein and a complete range of amino acids. They found that they were healthier while taking pollen. They could train longer and harder. The average daily run increased from 30 kilometers to 50 kilometers, an increase of 67%. They found that, during the winter season, they lost 77% fewer days to flu and cold illnesses than others who did not take pollen but took vitamins only.

During the 1968 Olympic Games in Mexico, the Finnish runners, normally very good at long distance running, failed to win any medals. As a result, their trainers began a specialized program of training and supplementing the training diet with Swedish pollen extract. They started to use pollen during the winter season training session of 1969-1970.

After two years of using pollen, Lasse Viren, the Finnish long distance runner, ran in the 10,000 meter race in the 1972 Olympic Games. By this time, he was in perfect condition and highly trained to the maximum level. During the race, he lost his balance and fell to the ground. He got up and, despite the large lead of the other runners, he had such immense power that he overtook them and won the Gold Medal. He still had enough energy at the end to run a victory lap, much to the delight of the spectators. It should be noted that the second place Silver Medal winner was also a Finnish runner by the name of Vassala.

Also in 1972, a symposium was held in Sweden detailing the positive effects of pollen extract. Three doctors from the professional football league in Italy reported on the use of pollen extract by nine of their football teams. Their report stated that the fatigue level was lowered from 12.75% to 3.75% after only ten days, and was lowered to zero after ninety days. Oxygen intake increased from 11.25% to 35%. The stamina test showed an increase from 13.75% to 36.2%. Fatigue was reduced, while oxygen intake and stamina was increased.

It is also rumored that Olympic coach Bella Karolyi gave pollen to his world-class gymnasts, including Nadia Comanech, Olga Korbut, Julie McNamara, and Mary Lou Retton. It is known for certain that pollen has been used by Muhammad

Ali, Olympic distance running champion Lasse Viren from Finland, and comedian-turned-health activist Dick Gregory.

Of the several Swedish pollen products available, a specific sports formula has been developed. It's an energy supplement used by professional athletes to increase capacity, strength and stamina in training and competition. It accelerates the transportation of nutrients to the cells, boosts vitality, speeds energy recovery time, fights fatigue, and expands anaerobic ability. It also works ideally as an energy pick-me-up during the day for anyone, athlete or non-athlete.

Pollen and Health

Clinics in dozens of countries have used Swedish pollen for a wide variety of conditions of ill health. Swedish courts actually stated that pollen extract was the only nutritional product in Sweden for which health claims could be made.

Twelve years ago, a large vitamin company for doctors published a book detailing nutritional therapy for health problems. Pollen extract was listed as the one recommended supplement that was common to virtually every condition in the book.

The key to optimal health is found within the metabolic processes of the body's cells — assimilation of nutrients and elimination of wastes. This is how the cell regenerates itself, continually building a new cell according to the genetic code of the RNA/DNA in the nucleus of the cell. Since Swedish pollen extract is the most perfect food for vitalizing cell functions, activating metabolism, and "feeding" genetic RNA/DNA replication according to the cellular blueprint, it is naturally the most perfect food for optimal health. It is truly the ultimate cell food.

In this regard, pollen is a glandular rocket fuel. The body's endocrine glands regulate all the systems of the body by secreting very small amounts of powerful hormones. Virtually all the precursors to these hormones are found within pollen extract. By supplying a full spectrum of all the essential micronutrients for cell metabolism and glandular function, Swedish pollen nurtures the self-regulatory functions of the

Swedish courts actually stated that pollen extract was the only nutritional product in Sweden for which health claims could be made.

body for stress management, weight control, and optimal health.

The natural benefit of optimal health is more energy. Pollen provides new vim, vigor, and vitality. Not only does the body have the wisdom to direct extra vital force and nutrients to any needy part of the body, but Swedish pollen extract allows the body to enjoy more of its vivacious feminine glow or powerful masculine virility by feeding all the cells, glands, and organs with what they need for vital energy.

Pollen also has a powerful antioxidant effect, as proven in the pollen research done by Dr. B.P. Poovaiah. Pollen helps deactivate or destroy free radicals created during the course of normal cellular activity, or those caused by smoking or eating dark roasted foods (coffee). It defends cells in vital organs against harmful effects caused by toxic substances in the environment and food.

The Swedish pollen company has developed a special product that contains pollen extract for a powerful pollen and antioxidant formula.

This is a synergistic formula blend containing antioxidants and detoxifying Swedish pollen extract. Pollen, when combined with antioxidants in this specialized formula, becomes a potent free radical eliminator, adding to our longevity and anti-aging plan. It neutralizes the activity of free radicals, slows the aging process in body and brain cells, and protects the skin against signs of early aging, wrinkles, pigmented spots, dryness, loss of tone and elasticity. It also improves the youthful appearance of hair and nails.

In addition, pollen extract appears to contain a group of components which are involved in helping the liver detoxify itself from harmful and toxic substances.

The main benefits of Swedish pollen are these: it supplies nutrients to the cells, boosts energy quickly, carries vitamins and minerals to the cell, acts as an antioxidant, helps the body adapt to stress, reduces platelet aggregation, helps stimulate the body's natural self-defense system, controls low serum lipid

In general, pollen maintains the reactivity and flexibility of the body and its functions and regulates the metabolic process and levels to maintain general well-being.

level, controls prostaglandin synthesis, and aids in liver detoxification.

In general, pollen maintains the reactivity and flexibility of the body and its functions and regulates the metabolic process and levels to maintain general well-being. It also helps control blood cholesterol and the function of the prostate.

Pollen has been used and studied in Europe for respiratory tract infections, appetite normalization in children and the elderly, reducing inflammations, nutrient assimilation in convalescent persons, reducing cholesterol levels, preventing or reducing hayfever, and as an immunostimulation inducer.

It enables better adaptation to stress, enhances physical and mental capacity, and gives added vitality and other long-lasting benefits with regular use.

Pollen has also been found to aid in both weight gain and weight loss. Apparently, it does this by normalizing the body's desire and use of digested food.

Pollen has also been found to aid in both weight gain and weight loss. Apparently, it does this by normalizing the body's desire and use of digested food.

Most amazing of all, Sir Alec Isaac, the Englishman who discovered interferon, studied pollen extract for two years. Interferon is the body's own natural disease fighting substance. The free amino acids in pollen extract are readily absorbed by the body, and are used by the body to build proteins such as interferon. Isaac found that pollen not only penetrates the wall of the cell, but also penetrates the cell membrane. It then combines with the cell RNA and DNA and synthesizes interferon for use by the body's immune system. Much scientific interest has arisen in interferon over the last few years for its use as a cancer treatment. It could be that pollen may have similar properties due to its interferon producing quality.

The History of Swedish Pollen Extract

The Swedish researcher who discovered pollen extract was a beekeeper, living in the southern region of Sweden. He developed a process to harvest pollen on a commercial scale to feed to his bees. This was not bee pollen that he was feeding them, but pure pollen collected directly from the plants by his own patented machinery. He found that by feeding the bees with his machine-collected pollen early in the year, the queen would lay more eggs, and the hive would produce more honey.

Even in these very beginning days of pollen research, he noted that his machine-collected pollen caused the queen bee to be more fertile. Years later, many human users of Swedish pollen would report that pollen allowed them to have more children, and seemed to increase the life span of both the sperm and egg cells. This one benefit may be a godsend to childless couples.

As research into the miracle of pollen continued, it was discovered that bees use it to make royal jelly. The royal jelly is fed to only one bee larvae, who later grows to be the queen of the colony. With three times the size, and ten times the life span of the other bees, the queen owes it all to one thing — a diet of highly synthesized pollen.

Excited by this, the researcher developed the original bee pollen trap, similar to those still used by beekeepers today. But he soon realized that he was robbing the bees of an essential food, pollen, while causing many bees to lose their legs or wings on the way through the trap. And he found a more serious problem with contaminants in the bee pollen.

Even today, bee pollen is graded by the amount of impurities such as bacteria, fungi, mites, rodent dung, fly eggs, and bee body parts found in it.

He then developed the world's only mechanical pollen harvester machine. An industrial secret to this day, this technology harvests tons of pollen every year.

But his research didn't stop there. He went on to discover how to remove the pollen food from the hard shell husk surrounding it. Bees, when making royal jelly, use their mandibles to crack and suck out the pollen food from inside the husk. For humans, the pollen husk is indigestible. So, people who are eating bee pollen aren't getting very much benefit because the pollen food is largely unavailable — only about 3% of the pollen can be digested from the hila opening on the side of the pollen grain. The remaining 97% of the pollen undigested and wasted.

Taking their cue from the bees, researchers developed a microbiological process to dissolve the membrane of the pollen husk, making the pure pollen food available for human digestion.

Taking their cues from the bees, the Swedish pollen researchers developed a microbiological process to dissolve the membrane of the pollen husk, making the pure pollen food available for human digestion.

The Swedish government tested pollen by giving it to soldiers in double blind tests. Pollen demonstrated effectiveness against both colds and flu in the harsh winter climates. Some inoperable tumors were treated with it and eliminated. Arthritis sufferers swore by it.

Professor Ask-Upmark, a Swedish physician, learned of Swedish pollen in 1957. He himself had suffered for several years from prostatitis. His wife convinced him to try the new pollen tablets to see if they would help him. His symptoms disappeared after only a short time. While away in England at a medical symposium, he forgot the pollen tablets. In only a few days, the old pain and inflammation had returned. He rushed home to Sweden, began taking pollen tablets again, and the symptoms disappeared in only four days.

He performed a test on ten prostatitis patients. Three of these ten men had been using other forms of therapy for five years with no improvement. After Professor Upmark treated them with pollen tablets, all ten men, 100%, became completely free of prostatitis symptoms.

CHART 9-2

Results of Double-Blind Studies in France with Swedish Flower Pollen

1. Decreased fatigue

2. Normalized weight and appetite

3. Increased hormone production in the body

4. Increased blood protein

5. Increased working capacity

6. Increased intellectual capacity

Dr. Leander, a urologist, tested 179 patients in a standard double-blind scientific test. He found that pollen tablets increased the recovery rate of his patients when compared to traditional treatments.

Dr. Vendel successfully used the pollen extract to treat measles and virus infections, such as colds and flu. He knew that the pollen helped the body to produce more interferon, a potent immune system substance.

There is a recorded case of a woman in Denmark who had been diagnosed with a rare disease called leucoencephalitis. There was no known treatment for this disease. The maximum life span after diagnosis is five years. No one had survived longer than that.

Tests in France showed that pollen was effective for use by anorexia sufferers. It was very nourishing and allowed them to normalize their weight.

CHART 9-3
Summary of the Benefits of Swedish Pollen Extract

- Stimulates body defense mechanisms.

- Produces an anti-inflammatory effect.

- Seems to induce an immunostimulation.

- Assists the immune system.

- Gives prolonged release of natural energy.

- Powers the ATP/ADP energy cycle.

- Antioxidant.

- Assists in cellular regeneration.

- Helps body release maximum amount of untapped energy from ATP cycle.

- 40 years of experience using this revolutionary technology.

At this time the woman was blind, paralyzed, almost deaf, and subject to as many as fifteen seizures a day. Her husband, quite by accident, met a doctor who heard of the wonderful Swedish pollen product. The husband began giving pollen to his wife. In fact, the Swedish pollen company agreed to supply the woman with ample supplies of pollen in both tablet and liquid form absolutely free for as long as she needed.

Slowly but surely, her health returned to her. Today, years later, this woman has regained her sight and hearing, can walk

---

CHART 9-4
Comments from Swedish Pollen Users:

- More positive mental outlook

- Increased feeling of well-being

- Less sleep required

- Higher energy levels

- Increased ability to accomplish work

- More alert

- Better athletic performance

- Improved digestion and nutrient assimilation

---

and do her own household chores. The pain and seizures have disappeared. She can visit her friends, and is happy and enjoys life. Her sole treatment consisted of pollen tablets and liquid pollen tonic. It can be hypothesized that the pollen boosted her body's systems in some way to relieve her very serious and life-threatening leucoencephalitis symptoms.

Tests in France showed that pollen was effective for use by anorexia sufferers. It was very nourishing and allowed them to normalize their weight. Pollen was registered in France for this use. Other double-blind studies in France showed that pollen had amazing results (see Chart 9-2).

In Japan, pollen is registered as a treatment for prostatitis.

In Poland, tests done by pharmacologists showed that pollen reduced harmful blood cholesterol by around 15%. It also reduced blood platelet aggregation. Blood aggregates can develop into blood clots and possibly cause heart attacks — pollen reduces this platelet aggregation. They studied the effect of pollen on the liver, and found that it had a protective effect against alcohols, carbon tetrachloride, and other toxins.

They also found that pollen had an anti-inflammatory quality, and suggested that the mechanism by which pollen reduces arterial plaque (anti-atherosclerotic) may be due to its polyunsaturated fatty acids and sterols which interfere with intestinal absorption of cholesterol.

In Germany, pollen is registered as a treatment for prostatitis. Researchers there found that pollen has a beneficial effect on cell metabolism. Dr. Habib also found that it had an effect on cancer cells in the prostate.

In Russia, pollen is registered as a treatment for prostatitis.

Over the last 35 years, Swedish researchers have led the world's first and best team of pollenologists to unlock the secrets of life stored in the entire food chain. Used by numerous Olympic champions and health conscious families in 52 countries of the world over the last 20 years, Swedish pollen extract has earned the reputation of nature's best food made better.

In Germany, pollen is registered as a treatment for prostatitis. Researchers there found that pollen has a beneficial effect on cell metabolism.

Appendix A

Reprinted with permission

UCLA Study Credits Vitamin C with 6 Year Life Extension

by Superfood Formulator Larry Meier

A long-term study began by UCLA scientists in 1971 analyzed vitamin C intake and the health of 11,348 adults.[1] The results of the study, published this past spring, indicated a 6 year increase in life-expectancy for men and a 1 year increase for women, consuming an average vitamin C supplement of 500 mg/day.

Men appear to benefit more due to vitamin C's preventative influence upon heart disease and stress related factors. This study clearly indicated that Vitamin C is far more important than most medical experts believed possible. The big questions now are, what form of vitamin C is best, and what synergistic factors best enable vitamin C's countermeasures against aging processes and disease? How much C is optimal and how many quality years can be added to your life?

There is, however, one thing that we can be absolutely certain about — Vitamin C, Pycnogenol and Bilberry will be among the antioxidant capsules taken with every meal and again at bedtime for yourself or your neighbor who wish to extend an active quality of life 5 to 20 years or more beyond the norm.

The other thing we know with full certainty is that you don't have to wait decades for this technology to arrive. It is available to you right now at reasonable cost, and it is never too late to start!

The UCLA study, while being very large and impressive in results, is already obsolete information. European scientists in Great Britain, France, Germany and Italy have raced to perfect a new generation of pro-vitamin C synergists that serve to better target and transport vitamin C to where it is needed. These synergists belong to the plant cell chemistry family of bioflavonoids, in a generally ignored branch of that family called **anthocyanadins ("Bilberry") and proanthocyanadins ("Pycnogenol")**. Concentrations are found in berries, grapes, pine cells and peanut skins. Pycnogenol lends peanut skins and some wines, their unique tart/bitter taste. The anthocyanadins lend blueberries and bilberry (English blueberry) their blue (cyan) color.

Stringent testing in Europe and centuries-long history of humans consuming these nutrients confirm their safety.

The English produce bilberry concentrate. The Italians extract theirs from peanut skins, and the Germans take theirs from grapes. The field is evolving rapidly, but at present, the German and English products seem to provide the most antioxidant power and benefit per nutrition dollar invested.

Of all the formulas and types of products I have worked with, next to the top on my list of favorites is the one where Vitamin C, Pycnogenol and Bilberry are combined. This unique synergistic blend delivers more vitamin C to the cellular sites where it is needed and then holds it there so it can get its protective and reconstructive work done.

Vitamin C is a unique nutrient that is essential for many functions within your body. Human beings are among the less than 1% of the animal kingdom that can't make their own Vitamin C. Based upon what animal bodies make for their daily needs, we should be producing or consuming 10,000 mg per day. But we don't. We are utterly dependent upon the Vitamin C content of our particular diet. The average intake is only 50 to 80 mg per day.

In addition to being an essential nutrient, Vitamin C is also a primary antioxidant. This is where the 60 mg RDA (recommended daily allowance) leaves us far short of an ideal intake. The RDA of vitamin C is a minimal amount necessary to prevent immediate and overt manifestations such as scurvy.

The RDA does not take any long-range antioxidant benefits into consideration. The more antioxidants flowing through your system, the slower toxins will damage your cells and their genetic blueprint — and the longer you will stay biologically young.

The manifestations of aging have as much to do with the amount of antioxidants you consume as they do with the clock. For some people, antioxidant supplements can even turn the clock back and hold it there for awhile, and, when it starts its inevitable pace, it will be at a much slower pace. A good program of antioxidants will keep you looking, feeling and performing younger than your mere chronological age. **Antioxidants provide both quantity AND quality of life.**

Every day that we age, we become more and more vulnerable to 3 primary killers — heart disease, cancer and infections.

A recent international conference of 130 scientists and physicians focused on 33 studies that found Vitamin C preventative to numerous types of cancer. One of the studies from the Linus Pauling Institute indicated one-fifth the rate of cancer with substantial intake of Vitamin C.

In a separate study, Dr. Eymard Poydock of Mercyhurst College in Erie, PA, noted that Vitamins C and B12 work together to form cobalt ascorbate which apparently **prevents division of tumor cells** without damaging normal cells.

In the book *Nutritional Influences on Illness*, Dr. Melvyn R. Werbach, M.D., reported an average 47 point drop in cholesterol to 181 within 6 weeks at 1,000 mg of Vitamin C daily. (A cholesterol level of 200 mg per decaliter is considered very good — 181 mg per decaliter would be regarded as excellent.) **The impact of this level of supplementation on heart disease, if followed by all Americans, would save hundreds of thousands of lives every year** and save countless others premature, expensive and miserable hospital or nursing home existence.

According to Dr. Raxit Jarewalla of the Linus Pauling Institute, Vitamin C suppresses the AIDS virus by **inhibiting viral replication in infected cells.** He noted that Vitamin C works at a different stage of the HIV life cycle from other treatments such as alpha-interferon.

Vitamin C is **also effective in bacterial infections** according to Abram Hoffer M.D., Ph.D., in his book *Orthomolecular Medicine for Physicians.* **It detoxifies bacterial toxins and helps to destroy invading substances.**

Dr. Richard Cutler of the National Institute on Aging's Gerontology Research Center in Baltimore is regarded by his peers as the scientist who may understand more about the physical forces behind cellular aging than any person alive. One of Dr. Cutler's more dramatic experiments indicated the level of total antioxidant protection in a variety of animals. **He concluded that humans are among the longest lived animals, not because of any single antioxidant, but because of our total combined antioxidants working together synergistically ("net antioxidant protection").** He concluded that life span may be a function of antioxidant set-points.

I believe that one of these primary "set-points" determining our life span is intercellular Vitamin C levels kept arbitrarily low because of Vitamin C's extreme water solubility. Like a fish trying to swim up a waterfall, vitamin C is continually being washed out of our systems in a very short period of time before it can reach optimal cellular saturation levels.

Throughout nature, Vitamin C is accompanied by substances called bioflavonoids. In my vitamin C formulation, I selected to combine the antioxidant bioflavonoids proanthocyanadins (Pycnogenol) and anthocyanadins (Bilberry) with 3 particularly bioavailable and buffered (low acid) forms of vitamin C as Calcium, Magnesium and Zinc Ascorbates.

This formulation assures optimal assimilation, without digestive upset (even at high levels of intake), along with assured delivery to, and holding power inside the cells where Vitamin C's antioxidant gene-protecting/cell-wall-protecting properties can do us the most life-extending good.

This same combination is also available as part of my complete superfood complex formula.

According to C-E's (a vitamin formula blend) co-designer, Nuclear Physicist, Health Enthusiast and Pycnogenol researcher, Dr. Hank Liers, Ph.D., Pycnogenol and Bilberry differ from other bioflavonoids in that they are extremely water soluble, highly bioavailable, nontoxic and nonmutagenic. **According to Nagasaki University School of Medicine, proanthocyanadins were shown to have an antioxidant effect 20 times greater than vitamin C and 50 times greater than Vitamin E.**

In addition, Dr. Liers states that proanthocyanadins possess significant collagen-stabilizing ability. Collagen is your body's most abundant protein, holding together everything from your skin and complexion to your muscles and ligaments. **Rheumatoid arthritis destroys collagen. Proanthocyanadins inhibit destruction of collagen by blocking certain products of inflammation.** Proanthocyanadins promote mucopolysaccharide biosynthesis and formation of new collagen. **(Mucopolysaccharides are also credited as being a prime active component of aloe vera.)**

Dr. Liers goes on to note that by inhibiting degradation of basement-membrane collagen of brain capillaries, proanthocyanadins help to restore and maintain the brain's protection from drugs, pollutants and toxins. Dr. Liers incorporates pycnogenol into his personal athletic program to minimize injury, enhance performance and reduce recovery time.

Vitamin C — Antidote To Mercury

With a developing awareness of mercury contamination from dental fillings, cosmetics, laxatives, fish and the environment — combined with the fact that it may take decades for half of the mercury you already have to leave your system, many people are wondering, what can be done with the mercury we already have?

A few of mercury's indicators include fatigue, chest pain, immune deficiency, irritability, moodiness, loss of memory, lack of concentration, depression, insomnia, digestive problems, vision and hearing impairment, dizziness, birth defects, tremor in fingers — and more. If experiencing any of these, seek professional care at once.

Dental fillings are 50% mercury. Every time you chew your food, some of the mercury is converted to a gas which you inhale. **The EPA forbids dentists from disposing of mercury filling particles down sewers, but does not prevent them from putting it in your mouth.** Authorities in Japan, Germany and Sweden are seriously considering full bans of mercury fillings. The EPA recently banned mercury from indoor paint. However, the mercury vapor level from your filled teeth after chewing may reach over 90 times the level of a newly painted room.

University of Calgary (Alberta Canada) Medical School professors Murray Vimy and Fritz Lorscheider put 12 fillings in the mouths of 6 sheep. Within one month all 6 lost 50% of their kidney function, an early indication of severe damage throughout other vital tissues.

In another study, European scientists Momcilo Mokranjae and Ceda Petrovic gave 20 guinea pigs 200 mg of vitamin C each for 6 days. Guinea pigs, like humans, do not make their own vitamin C and are utterly dependent upon dietary or supplemental vitamin C. On the sixth day, each animal was poisoned with a fatal level of mercury that should have killed them within a few hours. Vitamin C supplementation continued. After 20 days, all the animals were eating and behaving normally, and were considered saved and the experiment terminated.

Vitamin C is obviously one of the most effective cellular protectors and cleansers available. By combining Pycnogenol (antioxidant and Vitamin C carrier), Bilberry (antioxidant and Vitamin C holder/saver) with this vital antioxidant vitamin, you can enjoy optimal benefits from Vitamin C in every part of your body and every aspect of your life. When you benefit health on a cellular level, nothing escapes benefit and improvement — from energy to eyesight, to beauty and weight management, to sexuality and immunity.

Bilberry carries its own separate list of benefits including enhancement of night vision. In addition, European doctors use Pycnogenol and Bilberry as a treatment for varicose veins. **Isn't it time you started to take Vitamin C and its synergists seriously? You owe it to yourself to discover your personal best level of Vitamin C, Pycnogenol and Bilberry — Your personal** best level of health and performance.

REFERENCES

1. Enstrom JE, Kanim LE, Klein MA. "Vitamin C intake and mortality among a sample of the United States Population." EPIDEMIOLOGY. 1992; 3:194-202

2. C-E Vitamin C, Pycnogenol, Bilberry supplement is available from Quantum Advance International, Inc., 1336 S. 336 St. Federal Way, WA 98003-6348, (206) 874-9092 or 1-800-927-9336.

3. "Ascorbic Acid: Biological Functions and Relation to Cancer" Washington D.C., Fall of 1990, sponsored by National Cancer Institute and National Institute of Digestive and Kidney Diseases.

4. "Ascorbic Acid: Biological Functions and Relation to Cancer" as reported by HEALTH NEWS & REVIEW, Keats Publishing, JUL/AUG 1991.

5. "The 200-Year-Old-Man," LONGEVITY MAGAZINE, AUG 1992.

6. Exsula Ultima (see number 2 above).

7. THE LIFE ENTHUSIAST NEWSLETTER, Feb. 1991.

8. CBS News "60 MINUTES" December 16, 1990

9. Keats Publishing. Inc., HEALTH NEWS AND REVIEW, JUL/AUG, 1991, p. 17, "All That Glitters Is Not Silver," Jerome Mittleman, D.D.S.

10. C.R. ACAD. SC. PARIS, 1964 as reported in Rodale, ed., PREVENTION, JUL 1972, p. 82

Appendix B

Reprinted with Permission

Seven Key Energies of Life and Longevity

by Superfood Formulator Larry Meier

1 **CALORIC ENERGY** comes primarily from carbohydrates and lipids (fats). This is the energy necessary to keep you warm, thinking and in motion. This is chemical energy for your body like gasoline is fuel for your car.

Excellent sources of caloric energy include **clean-burning** high quality carbohydrates (sugars, starches and fiber) as found in natural fruits, grains and vegetables.

SPIRULINA is an excellent source of a rare carbohydrate called **rhamnose**. This carbohydrate is especially favored by athletes for **exceptional stamina**. Similar carbohydrates are found in **CHLORELLA**.

Other plant carbohydrates such as those in **GREEN WHEAT and BARLEY GRASS JUICE** are renowned for their "horse power" and stamina they provide oxen and race horses. As a result, the juices from these plants are also favored by many athletes.

ROYAL JELLY and BEE POLLEN carbohydrates fire the incredibly ambitious honey bees. These foods are the super fuels of nature refined by the bees from the pollen, or life essence of flowers. These are also a favorite of athletes and intellectual top achievers.

APPLE FIBER is a source of high quality fiber which can be converted to energy. However, energy is a minor role. Fiber's primary purpose is to aid intestinal action and proper elimination.

SOYBEAN LECITHIN provides your liver with excellent lecithin resources. Your liver manufactures lecithin from food lecithins, fats and minerals. **LECITHIN** is perhaps the finest practical source of essential fatty acids available. Once lecithin has completed its other tasks in the body — such as dissolving cholesterol, fueling creativity and supporting beautiful healthy skin — it goes on to be consumed as a quality source of carbohydrates and lipids providing fuel for physical and mental activity.

Poor sources of sugars and fats are those "refined" foods which have had many of their natural nutrient factors and enzymes compromised during processing. If certain nutrients and enzymes are absent, proper carbohydrate and lipid metabolism cannot take place, and the intricate machinery of life becomes fouled and malfunctions. Diets with even small amounts of refined sugars and fats can result in disproportionately high weight gain as the system becomes clogged. The cholesterol factor and excessive protein content of meat and dairy products makes them an especially unhealthy source of fats. An impressive amount of research links meat and dairy products, along with an overabundance of refined fats and sugars, to a smorgasbord of health problems ranging from high blood pressure to diabetes, overweight and osteoporosis.

2 **AMBITION ENERGY** is a combined quality of a ready, healthy body available to a positive thinking mind. When your body feels good, you are more likely to feel ambitious. When your body is heavy and feeling poorly, that is a definite impediment to ambition. A healthful nutritious diet, providing plant-grown vitamins, minerals and enzymes, supports important ambition resources.

LECITHIN and COENZYME Q10 are favorites for contributing to feeling capable and for supporting a positive spirit of ambition. Whether for students, housewives, blue collar workers or professionals, quantity and quality of work output is directly related to quality of nutritional input.

3 **MENTAL ENERGY** must compete with physical energy for your body's limited physical resources. If physical exertion is extreme, reserves for mental energy will suffer and vice versa. Balance and moderation in your lifestyle is essential for optimal health and longevity. And so is a plentiful supply of certain key nutrients.

LECITHIN is a perfect source of the B vitamin choline. Choline is a resource used by your body to make acetylcholine, the primary neurotransmitter. Your brain operates on chemical-electrical principles. When thought takes place, neurotransmitter chemicals are transformed and used up in the transmission of nerve signals. A plentiful reserve of lecithin can help support the extra mental capacity, clarity and memory necessary to cope with the stresses and challenges of a fast-paced world.

VITAMIN C is approximately 100 times more concentrated in the brain as elsewhere in your body. Special tiny vitamin C pumps along the spinal chord and in your head make this possible. This system assures a plentiful supply of the antioxidant vitamin C is available to protect these especially vulnerable and important cells from the metabolic toxins of body energy production as well as pollutant chemicals from the outside as found if in food, air and beverages.

4 **SEXUAL ENERGY** is highly dependent upon certain key nutrients.

VITAMIN E is so important for sexual health that it has actually been called the "sex vitamin" by some researchers and enthusiasts. Vitamin E is a powerful antioxidant that protects cells from toxins, thus resulting in a deep overall sense of well-being. Feeling well is a prerequisite to feeling romantic. The body also uses vitamin E as an essential nutrient. The nutritional needs for vitamin E are quite low, probably less than 20 IU per day. The antioxidant opportunities are much greater. Many enthusiasts take upwards of 1000 IU per day for optimal antioxidant benefits.

LECITHIN is equal in sexual benefit to vitamin E. For women, lecithin is an important component of natural lubrication. For men, it is of value to help replace lecithin lost with their semen.

Sound, overall nutrition is essential to support the feelings of well-being and self-esteem so vital to a fulfilling romantic life.

5 CLEANSING ENERGY is supported by antioxidant nutrients and enzymes as well as the accessory nutrient chlorophyll.

CHLOROPHYLL is the green pigment lending its color to most of the plant life on our planet. Though its abundance hints at its importance, it is remarkably scarce in our modern diets. Among natural healing practitioners, chlorophyll is highly regarded as a most powerful body cleanser, deodorizer and purifier. **SPIRULINA, CHLORELLA and WHEAT & BARLEY GRASS JUICE** are especially rich sources of chlorophyll.

ANTIOXIDANT ENZYMES are produced by our bodies from nutrients in our foods. They keep our cells clean and youthful. SOme antioxidant enzymes are produced by plant cells in an effort to protect genetic material and help clear toxins out of the intricate cells. According to natural food enthusiasts, certain uncooked fresh or carefully dehydrated herbs, grasses, fruits, vegetables, along with sprouting grains and seeds, can be counted upon to provide these enzymes in a ready to use form.

SUPEROXIDE DISMUTASE and COENZYME Q10 are 2 of the most highly prized antioxidant enzymes. An effective superfood blend will contain outstanding concentrations of these and many other valuable antioxidant enzymes. A properly designed and balanced formulation will attend to their effective assimilation.

6 HEALING ENERGY will either happen or not happen depending upon many different nutrients. Enzymes, antioxidants, and clean, high quality proteins, along with virtually every known nutrient are acknowledged to play some role. Many who have been victorious over cancer and other challenges to their health, attribute their newfound health to consuming a vegetarian diet rich in an abundance of raw fruit and vegetable juices and sprouts, along with a variety of superfoods and nutritional supplements.

With all of the mounting evidence and countless personal victories, certainly no objective researcher or sincere practitioner would oppose a healthful diet, along with substantial nutritional supplementation as an essential part of an y serious healing regimen.

VITAMINS A (CAROTENE) C and E are generally recognized to the the 3 most important vitamins for healing.

Harvard University research and over a dozen other major studies found dietary carotene crucial in supporting your body's resistance to the daily assault by cancer-causing substances. The types of carotenes found in plant cells can be converted by your body into an amazing substance called Tumor Necrosis Factor Alpha. Your immune system uses TNF Alpha to destroy invaders and mutant cells. Obviously, with growing environmental pollution abounding, one could reasonably conclude that your intake of foods rich in carotene should be especially abundant.

DUNALIELLA ALGAE (a microscopic sea plant) is an incredibly great source of carotenes. **SPIRULINA, CHLORELLA and KLAMATH ALGAES** are nearly as rich. A single gram of any one of these super plants can easily contain more carotene than many Americans will eat in a week. Even a green-vegetable-loving vegetarian can feel more secure in a carcinogen-filled world by adding a serving of these carotene-rich super plants to their daily diet.

7 LONGEVITY ENERGY is proportional to certain antioxidant resources "left over at the end of the day" to invest in preservation after all the essential chores in the cells are done.

Increasingly, researchers are compelled to admit that nutrient levels considered for years to be adequate in preventing malnutrition are just that — merely adequate — not optimal! Longevity, commonly thought of as exceptional quality and quantity of life is dependent upon exceptional nutrient and antioxidant resources.

This is logical when you consider the premature aging manifestations of someone suffering malnutrition — such as prisoners of war in WWII, Europe and Japan, or later in Vietnam, or present day Africa or Bangladesh. In these cases it becomes much more obvious that velocity of biological aging is proportional to dietary quality.

No thinking person would willingly write and sign a statement saying they wished for their lives to decline and expire at an average age. Yet few are compelled to take even the most convenient and economical measures now to impact something hoped to be years or decades away.

COENZYME Q10, VITAMINS A, C and E, CAROTENE (PLANT SOURCED VITAMIN A) and certain botanical compounds and antioxidant enzymes in **GINKGO BILOBA, green and blue berries (PYCNOGENOL and BILBERRY EXTRACT) SUMA, HIGH TRANSFERULIC RICE BRAN, MILK THISTLE, ROYAL JELLY, CHLORELLA, SPIRULINA, WHEAT & BARLEY GRASS JUICE,** comprise a virtual who's who of the antioxidant superstars.

Many longevity and health enthusiasts are already taking these superfoods separately without realizing what a high total dollar amount they are actually paying. For anyone interested in preserving or optimizing their life, a top quality superfood blend is a more economical way to go.

Stresses, over-processed foods, seriously depleted soils and poor eating habits are causing millions to lose their desire and zest for life. Superfood blends are the best way I know of getting all of the important accessory nutrients, trace minerals, enzymes and other beneficial supportive factors that your body so desperately needs for empowering these seven key energies and making your life the longest and best that it can be.

Appendix C

Reprinted with permission

Antioxidant Enzymes: Avenues of Activity

by Superfood Formulator Larry Meier

Questions and Answers

A collection of the toughest and most interesting questions I've been asked.

Question: I feel that a person who takes supplements is experimenting with themselves. Isn't it all too good to be true? It seems the entire concept is some invention of modern marketing.

Answer: *Old age must be resisted and its deficiencies supplied* - Cicero, 50 B.C.

The famous scientist Michael Faraday once said, *"Nothing is too wonderful to be true."* Of course that doesn't mean that everything that's cracked up to be wonderful is wonderful. All it means is that just because something is wonderful doesn't automatically mean it isn't true. The most dangerous experiments are the ones we participate in unconsciously ... *"Since we make them without knowing it, we are powerless to abandon them."* - Henri Poincare

Question: Every now and then someone sends me a newspaper clipping quoting some nutritionist saying that barley juice is a waste of money, because enzymes like SOD can't survive the stomach acids. I've been getting good results from barley juice for years. Whenever I stop taking it, all sorts of old aches and pains return. But, I am confused by the contradictory information from the experts.

Answer: Be careful of how you stand in awe before these nutritionists. Consider that these are the same people whose years in college trained them that jello is an indispensable part of every hospital menu. Someone has to challenge convention, otherwise we'd still be blood-letting for pneumonia. Effectiveness is what counts – what works for you! Let's talk about superoxide dismutase (SOD), pronounced like "sawed".

SOD is a very beneficial antioxidant enzyme now receiving lots of press. Dangerously reactive molecular oxygen (O_2 containing an unpaired electron) is produced throughout the cells of your body trillions of times a second as a by-product of the conversion of food and oxygen to life energy.

Unless it is defused, this highly destructive superoxide form of oxygen can literally zap holes in your genetic blueprints. When cellular blueprints become defective they will not be able to replicate themselves accurately, resulting in signs of aging, disease and cancer.

Superoxide dismutase "dis-mutates" (reverses the mutation of) the destructive superactive unpaired electron state of these O_2 molecules.

Accordingly, a study by biophysicist, Dr. Richard Cutler at the National Institute of Aging, found that the life spans of man and many other mammals is directly proportional to the SOD content in their heart, brain and liver!

Your body obtains precious SOD from 2 sources — preformed SOD in some raw foods, and bodily produced SOD constructed mostly in your liver from the simpler food elements, amino acids and minerals. Your liver attaches a beneficially active life force to this complex molecule. Your liver's SOD production declines from about 1,700 units per gram of body weight to less than 50 units per gram at age 80. This is why consumption of foods rich in SOD will become ever more important to you as you age.

Four exceptional food sources of SOD have been discovered and stabilizing methods perfected. They are: Spirulina (a microscopic sea vegetable), green wheat and barley grass juices, and sprouting seeds. My formula is the only food concentrate to contain SOD from all four.

The SOD used in original medical research was an unstable SOD isolated from horse blood and beef liver. It had to be injected directly into the blood stream to get the desired results. The vegetable sources of SOD mentioned above have produced "miraculous" benefits when taken orally, as if your Creator designed these foods to deliver SOD to your body. The other nutrients and enzymes in these foods work synergistically to enhance the effectiveness of SOD and encourage its increased production by your body.

SEARCHING FOR THE KEYS...
...IN THE RIGHT PLACE

The experimentor who does not know what he is looking for will not understand what he finds.

— Claude Bernard, 1813-1878

Japanese scientists have discovered that the antioxidant enzyme relative of SOD, peroxidase P4D1 leaps into a much higher state of activity when exposed to the acidic environment of the stomach (Kazuhiko Kubota, Ph.D.).

Incredibly, it is as if P4D1 were designed to be a watch-dog awakening exactly there for the specific purpose of protecting humans from the nitric compounds that comprise the great majority of cancer causing chemicals that we are exposed to. Fried, charred and roasted foods and beverages (coffee) can contain up to 20,000 times the carcinogenicity of the benzopyrine and alkaloids in cigarette smoke! The tens of thousands of Americans dying of cancer of the stomach and colon each year indeed indicate that this is an all important battle field against cancer where antioxidant enzymes are quite beneficial. Vegetarians consuming fewer fired meats and more raw vegetable enzymes enjoy a greatly decreased incidence of cancers. If these toxins are allowed to pass through to the intestine without being deactivated, then your body is going to have to find an antidote to their cancer instigating activity that will be thoroughly effective in every possible environment and cell of the body - or, all types of cancer will ensue.

The argument is made that because enzyme molecules are highly complex, they are vulnerable to destruction - "stomach acid leaves them devoid of any activity." The remarkable activities of the antioxidant enzyme P4D1 reside within a molecule with a molecular weight of 53,000! Structurally, comparing this to the simpler molecules of vitamins, it's like the difference between a blow dryer and the space shuttle. Yet, P4D1's activities thrive in the very environment that is supposed to rip it apart. It's the decrease in nitric compounds that is important. Remaining enzymes chase escaping cancer starters into the lymphatic ducts where they continue to blow each other away, if they are doing their respective jobs.

Furthermore, stomach acid also activates the digestive enzymes that are so vital to digestion. Again, this is an example of enzyme activity designed to thrive in the environment of the stomach. If these particular enzymes become activated before leaving the pancreas it causes pancreatitis, an inflamed self-digestion. I wonder how many pancreases evolution digested before it got these enzymes in the proper place? Should I be disappointed that these particular enzymes are put to work in my gut and not in my blood stream?

EVIDENCE OF THE EFFECTIVENESS OF ENZYMES TAKEN ORALLY IS BEGINNING TO OVERWHELM SKEPTICS
- Dr. Peter Rothschild

Question: But, can food concentrates actually deliver usable SOD to the body, and if so, what are the potential benefits?

Answer: According to Dr. Mary Ruth Swope, a sparkling health enthusiast, in her book Green Leaves of Barley, *"Dried barley juice is an excellent natural source of SOD."* And, according to Dr. Yoshihide Hagiwara, M.D., winner of Japan's most prestigious science award for his work with food enzymes, *"these enzymes are absorbed directly through membranes in the mouth,*

throat and stomach ..." "... more effective when sipped rather than gulped down."

Peter R. Rothschild, M.D., Ph.D., Biochemist and Quantum Physicist, nominated for the Nobel Prize in Physics and author of 16 scientific books, based his work on enzymes on studies performed in West Germany, Switzerland, Italy, Mexico and Austria. His new research has found that even the largest enzyme molecules like SOD, catalases and peroxidases, *"taken orally in coated or uncoated form prior to meals,"* do survive in significance all the way to the bloodstream — 1 hour after consumption. In a recent study he even demonstrated the avenue of absorption as being via enzyme molecule bonding with emulsifying lipids (lecithin) into a *"liposome which has practically no surface tension and can thus penetrate the venules of the mucous and submucous layers to the lymphatic receptors located under the muscle layer of the intestines."*

By blending lecithin with the enzyme concentrates in my superfood formula we are favoring this critical enzyme to liposome conversion for the highest possible assimilation. This is the only formula on the market to combine high potency enzyme concentrates with lecithin for greatly enhanced results.

As for other potential benefits of antioxidant enzymes, Kazuhiko Kubota, Ph.D., Research Biologist and Specialist in Genetic Engineering at the University of California, San Diego, is pointing to SOD as an effective stimulant of repair of damaged DNA, especially when combined with the peroxidase P4D1 of cereal grass juice. Together, these enzymes have been observed to multiply by several fold better the cells' abilities to repair their own DNA! No other substances are known to have this incredible ability to stimulate repair of the blueprint of life!

LIFE IS ENZYMES

Nobel laureate James B. Sumner of Cornell University defined life as an orderly functioning of enzymes. Life ends when the worn-out metabolic activity of the body machine drops to such a low point that it is unable to carry on vital enzyme reactions. If we postpone the debilitation of metabolic enzyme activity, what we now call old age could become the glorious prime of life. Humans' enzymeless diets use up a tremendous amount of enzyme potential. The result is a short lived lifespan, illness, and lowered resistance to stresses of all types.

The length of life is directly proportional to the rate of exhaustion of the enzyme potential of an organism. The increased use of food enzymes promotes a decreased rate of exhaustion of the enzyme potential.

By eating foods with their enzymes intact... we can stop abnormal and pathological aging processes.

- Edward Howell M.D., Pioneering Biochemist and Nutrition Researcher, Enzyme Nutrition, 1985.

We were all hearty seamen, no colds did we fear,
And we have from all sickness entirely kept clear.
Thanks be to the Captain, he has proved so good
Amongst all the Islands to give us fresh food.
- From a 1700's sailor's song

Inhibition of Thiobarbituric Acid Reactive Products in Rat Liver Homogenate by Extracts from Pollen Grains

B.P. Poovaiah & S.T. Omaye

[Proc. West. Pharmacol. Soc. 30:67-69 (1987)]

Pollen grains or extracts prepared from pollen grains have been used as a food source or as a food supplement since the time of Hippocrates. Proponent claims have been cited for the use of such materials to improve health. Pollen extracts have been reported to have lipid lowering effects in animals (1,2) and in humans (3,4) fed high fat diet, decreased platelet aggregation (4), delayed appearance of mammary tumors in mice (5) and inhibition of carbon tetrachloride induced liver damage (6). Since investigations suggest a relationship exists between lipid metabolism and the ingestion of pollen, we conducted the following preliminary study to determine the antioxidant properties of extracts isolated from pollen grains <u>in vitro</u>. We also determined the LD_{50} of pollen grain extracts in mice.

<u>METHODS</u>: The lipid soluble fraction (GBX) and water soluble (T60) fraction extracted from pollen grains were tested for their ability to inhibit the formation of thiobarbituric acid reactive products (TBARP) or the chloroform extractable conjugated diene (CD). Both TBARP and CD may be initiated by the addition of carbon tetrachloride to rat liver homogenate. Homogenate of rat livers were prepared in isotonic Tris-buffer (0.25 M), pH 7.4. The homogenates were centrifuged at 10,000 x g for 20 minutes at 5° C and the supernatant (liver extracts) were saved on ice for the tests. In a total volume of 10 ml, the final concentrations were 0.05 or 0.5% for the antioxidant alpha-tocopherol or for the pollen extracts of GBX or T60. Carbon tetrachloride (an initiator of lipid peroxidation) was added to liver extract at the final concentration of 2 mM. After incubation at 37°C for various time periods, duplicate aliquots were removed and the reaction stopped by adding trichloroacetic acid (10%) containing 2-thiobarbituric acid (0.8%). The samples were placed in a boiling water bath for 10 minutes, cooled, centrifuged at 1,400 x g for 15 minutes and the colored product was measured at 532nm (7). This method measured TBARP that either were initially present or had evolved under the conditions of the test.

After 2 h of incubation at 37°C, aliquots of liver homogenate were extracted with chloroform:methanol (2:1) for CD. The extracted CDs of lipid peroxidation were dried under nitrogen, resuspended in cyclohexane and measured at 233 nm (8).

Acute oral toxicity of GBX and T60 were done in young adult male Sprague-Dawley rats. The test materials GBX

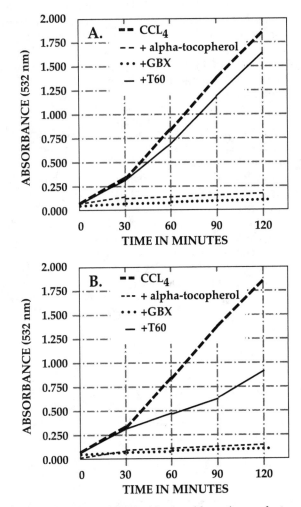

FIGURE 1: Inhibition of thiobarbituric acid-reactive products (TBARP) in rat liver homogenate by alpha-tocopherol, GBX and T60. A. 0.05% final concentration for alpha-tocopherol, GBX and T60. B. 0.5% final concentration for alpha-tocopherol, GBX and T60. Each point represents the mean of 2 determinations.

and T60 were administered undiluted at dosages of 20, 12.6, 7.9 and 5 g/kg to four groups of 5 rats. Animals were observed for gross signs of toxicity and death for 14 days. At the end of 14 day observation period, the rats were weighed, killed, and given a gross necropsy.

RESULTS. Fig. 1 summarizes the data regarding the effect of GBX and T60 on the formation of TBARP (increased absorbance at 532 nm) in rat liver homogenate. The inhibition of TBARP was dependent on the concentration of either alpha-tocopherol, GBX or T60. From this preliminary experiment, GBX was found to be as potent as alpha-tocopherol in the prevention of TBARP formation. T60 was much less effective in the inhibition of carbon tetrachloride initiated TBARP formation (about 10 to 55% as effective).

Lipid peroxidation, as determined by CDs, was reduced 18.9, 12.3, and 14.1% by .05% alpha-tocopherol, 0.05% GBX, and 0.5% T60 respectively in a liver homogenate incubated for 2 h.

Acute oral toxicity of GBX and T60 was found to be greater than 20 g/kg in male Sprague-Dawley rats. These results suggest that pollen grain extracts can inhibit lipid peroxidation and are not acutely toxic by oral administration in rats.

DISCUSSION: The thiobarbituric acid-reactive product (TBARP) test is one of the more commonly used methods for the detection of lipid peroxidation (9). However, like many biochemical methods, the popularity of a method is not in itself ultimate proof. Condensation occurs between two molecules of thiobarbituric acid and one molecule of malonaldehyde. Malonaldehyde is a by-product of lipid peroxidation. Conjugated diene measurements provide an alternative to the TBARP index, but is not conclusive either. These results suggest that lipid peroxidation can be inhibited by GBX and, perhaps, to lesser extent by T60 in an in vitro system containing a known propagate of lipid damage. It would be valuable to determine whether other indices of lipid peroxidation, either in vitro or in vivo, are inhibited by GBX and T60.

The acute toxicity of GBX and T60 were found to be greater than 20 g/kg in male Sprague-Dawley rats. Therefore, the pollen grain extracts are not classified toxic by oral administration.

ACKNOWLEDGEMENT: The Hilltop Research Inc., Cincinnati, Ohio, for the LD_{50} determination of GBX and T60 in rats.

REFERENCES
1. Samochowiec, L. & Wojeicki, J.: Herba Polon. 29:333 (1981).
2. Samochowiec, L. & Wojeicki, J.: Herba Polon. 29:165 (1983).
3. Wojeicki, J., Kosmider, K., Samochowiec, L. & Woyke, M.: Herba Polon. 29:56 (1983).
4. Kosmider, K., Wojeicki, J., Samochowiec, L., Woyke, M. & Gornik, W.: Herba Polon. 29:237 (1983).
5. Robinson, W.: J. Natl. Canc. Inst. 9:119 (1948).
6. Wojeicki, J. & Samochowiec, L.: Herba Polon. 30:1 (1984).
7. Reddy, K.A., Litov, R.E. & Omaye, S.T.: Res. Commun. Chem. Pathol. Pharmacol. 17:87 (1977).
8. Gray, J.I.: J. Amer. Oil Chem. Soc. 55:539 (1978).
9. Reddy, K.A. & Omaye, S.T.: In Inhalation Toxicology. (ed) II, Salem, Marcel Dekker, New York, 1985, p. 223.

Reprinted with permission

Silent Sufferers — Prostate Problems Affect 50% of Men over 50

Prostabrit Press Release

Half of all men over 50 suffer symptoms of enlargement of the prostatic gland, "Benign Prostatic Hyperplasia" (BPH), thought to be due to hormonal changes in advancing years.

Symptoms of BPH including discomfort during urination, frequent nocturnal micturition, hesitancy, dribbling, and the feeling of incomplete bladder void. While most men do not experience tremendous pain, it is a nuisance and can become socially embarrassing as time goes on.

If the impairment and discomfort caused by the growth of the prostate becomes too great, the standard treatment is surgery, and a prostatectomy is performed to remove the superfluous prostatic tissue.

At present there are an estimated 50,000 men in the UK awaiting surgery, with delays said to be between 18-24 months. A prostatectomy necessitates 5 days hospitalisation and a substantial convalescence.

In recent years evidence has been growing in support of alternative natural management of BPH. Pharmacological studies and clinical trials have shown ProstaBrit, a natural non-allergenic formulation of pollen extracts, to have significant therapeutic effects in cases of BPH, by its inhibitory nature on inflammation and oedema on prostatic tissue.

The clinical papers show that taken daily, ProstaBrit provided symptomatic relief from frequent micturition and reduced the residual urinary volume.

In other European countries ProstaBrit is available on prescription and as an over the counter preparation, and toxicology studies and clinical trials have confirmed its low incidence of side effects.

ProstaBrit can now be obtained directly from Health Products (in Europe) at $40.00 for one months' supply.

BENIGN PROSTATIC HYPERTROPHY

As part of the aging process in man, the prostate gland, over the age of 45 years, undergoes a condition of benign glandular and muscular hypertrophy. The result is an obstruction to the flow of urine and poor emptying of the bladder. In addition, it causes a disturbance in the neurological control of the bladder leading to irritative functional symptoms. BPH (benign prostatic hypertrophy), as it is called, is the single most frequent disease dealt with in urological practice. The treatment is surgical removal of the obstructive elements of the gland either by transurethral resection or rarely, these days, by open operation. Clearly, with an increasingly aging population the problem is set to worsen and this has both medical resource and economic implications.

At the present time, approximately 35,000 prostate operations are performed annually in the UK and ten times that number in the USA, at a staggering cost of more than 1 billion dollars. It is estimated that about 50,000 patients in the UK are awaiting operation. In recent years there has been considerable interest in alternative modalities of treatment, if not as a definitive cure then as an interim measure to relieve the symptoms particularly in patients with early signs of the disease.

As the prostate gland is a secondary sex gland, its growth and function is under hormonal control. Thus, one group of drugs that have been used to shrink the prostate gland are the inhibitors of the male hormone system. Another group are drugs that block the neurological pathways of bladder and prostate innervation, in an attempt to relieve the irritative symptoms. Unfortunately, these drugs have unpleasant and undesirable side effects, particularly in the elderly. Throughout Europe and the Far East, the use of extracts from herbs and plants, under licence, have been extensively employed to treat patients with mild or moderate symptoms of BPH. In this group the common agents are Permixon, derived from the American dwarf palm, Tadenan from the African prune, and Harzol from the root of Hypoxis rooperi. An extract of pollen has been in use for prostatic disease for over 20 years. It was first indicated in the use of prostatic inflammatory disease, a common condition in the younger male, but more recent clinical studies in several hundred patients in several centres in Europe and the UK indicate that it is as effective as all other forms of medication, including prostate hyperthermia, in relieving the symptoms of BPH, and has the advantage of being free from side effects.

Dr. C. Buck F.R.C.S.
Glasgow Royal Infirmary

The Cellular Aging Process and Free Radicals

by Pierre Carlotti, Sederma, France and Denise Gabrielle, Sederma, Inc.

Cutaneous aging, inevitable but a process of major concern, is being continuously researched to better understand the biological mechanism involved. Much of this research has attributed light and oxygen roles in the destruction of cellular membranes and the aging of the organism. UV radiation and oxidation reactions are continuously causing the formation of free radicals, which being highly reactive, cause inactivation and destruction of phospholipids along with other components of the cellular membrane. Therefore these highly reactive molecules must be removed as quickly as possible, since failure to do so is likely to lead to accumulation which would increase rate of damage. (1)

Various studies support this theory, attributing the relationship of lipid peroxides (or more specifically, free radicals) to inflammatory diseases and cancers. Today, we know that free radicals derived from oxygen, such as the hydroxyl radical

$$(\,^{\bullet}OH\,)$$

Superoxide anion

$$(O_2^{\bullet -})$$

and also singlet oxygen, along with the lipidic peroxidation phenomenon, play a significant role in cellular biology and consequently the cutaneous aging process. Free radicals, being atoms or molecules possessing one or more unpaired electrons, are usually represented by the symbol

$$R^{\bullet}$$

and develop as a result of absorption of energy, sufficient to rupture a covalent bond.

$$R:H \xrightarrow{\text{ENERGY}} R^{\bullet} + H^{\bullet}$$

Once formed, free radicals are extremely unstable, having strong tendency to pair up their electrons, turning them into powerful aggressors, thus causing them to set off chain reactions that make them self propagating.

$$R^{\bullet} + H\text{-}X \longrightarrow R\text{-}X + X^{\bullet}$$

However, free radicals formed from polyunsaturated molecules are stabilized by a molecular rearrangement of a conjugated diene, making them even more reactive.

Due to its association in formation of lipid peroxides and free radicals, oxygen obviously has an indirect negative effect, strongly influencing the longevity of cell life. In addition, the ubiquitousness of iron and oxygen in living organisms creates favorable conditions for formation of free radicals (Reaction 1), which also is accelerated by the following: (1) light and ionizing radiation, (2) agents such as glutathion and ascorbate that progressively reduce the oxygen molecule; (3) the "respiratory burst," a pathological phenomenon found during inflammation. The first of these are important stimulators in forming free radicals, since they not only increase the energy supply of oxygen, but when light and ionizing radiation are absorbed by photosensitive molecules, such as organic molecules, promote electrons to higher orbitals. These electrons now are more loosely bound than those of the ground state, thus causing them to be more easily abstractable by oxidizing agents. Therefore, when a photosensitive molecule is in the presence of atmospheric oxygen and light, the superoxide anion is formed. (2)

$$R + h\sqrt{} \longrightarrow (R^{+} + e^{-}) \xrightarrow{O_2} (R^{+} + O_2^{\bullet -})$$

It is believed that this superoxide anion favors formation of the OH radical, first by its transformation to H_2O_2, which then may be catalized by the presence of iron to form the hydroxyl radical.

$$\text{LIGHT} + \begin{array}{c}\text{PHOTOSENSITIVE}\\ \text{MOLECULE}\end{array} \xrightarrow{O_2}$$

$$O_2^{\bullet -} \longrightarrow H_2O_2 \xrightarrow{Fe_2^{+}} {}^{-}OH$$

REACTION 1: Formation of OH Radical

The OH radical is an extremely reactive molecule, considered one of the most "dangerous" of the free radicals, its main target being lipids but more specifically polyunsaturated fatty acids. It also attacks cholesterol, proteins, hyaluronic acid, nucleic acids and other components of the cellular membrane.

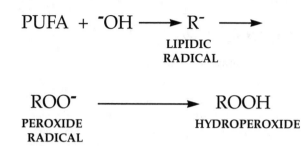

$$PUFA + \cdot OH \longrightarrow R^- \longrightarrow$$

LIPIDIC RADICAL

$$ROO^- \longrightarrow ROOH$$

PEROXIDE RADICAL   HYDROPEROXIDE

REACTION 2: Chain Reaction of Polyunsaturated Fatty Acids

Nowadays, numerous free radical scavengers (for example vitamin E, S.O.D., beta carotene, tannins, gingko biloba, selenium) are well known. However, it shouldn't be forgotten that under certain conditions — chemical environment or concentration of the scavenger — some actually may promote the formation of free radicals. Keeping this in mind, after two years of research, Sederma has launched a new product called Iniferine(5) designed to fight more efficiently against free radicals, particularly the OH radical. This is a natural enzymatic anti-free radical complex containing three very stable molecules found in biological fluids, which function as follows:

First, lactoferrin, a highly soluble natural glycoprotein, stable in aqueous solution, with a molecular weight of approximately 70,000 Daltons, is capable of binding to two ferric ions (Fe^{3+}) per molecule, therefore limiting the formation of the OH radical through reaction 1. Second, 2-thioxanthine, a natural odorless white powder capable of trapping all types of free radicals due mainly to the function of its thiol (SH).

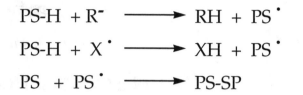

$$PS\text{-}H + R^- \longrightarrow RH + PS\cdot$$
$$PS\text{-}H + X\cdot \longrightarrow XH + PS\cdot$$
$$PS + PS\cdot \longrightarrow PS\text{-}SP$$

Third, 8-hydroxyxanthine, also a natural white powder, can trap the OH radical and neutralize singlet oxygen by formation of allantoin.

To prove the strong activity of **Iniferine**, a biological model was used to test numerous anti-free radical preparations. This in vitro test was performed on soy phospholipid liposomes, due to their high level of poly-unsaturated fatty acids (PUFA). Free radicals attack these liposomes causing peroxidation of the PUFA, leading to generation of conjugated dienes. It is possible to evaluate the anti-free radical power of a preparation by measuring these conjugated dienes by the use of UV spectrophotometry at 233 mm. This leads to the conclusion that this material is an effective, safe way of preventing damage and inactivation of biological molecules caused by free radicals — thus preventing aging, especially that due to solar exposure.

REFERENCES
1. Kanungo, M.S., "Biochemistry of Ageing," Academic Press, London, 1980.
2. Author, A.P. (Editor), Foote, C.S. (Ch.10): Del Maestro, R.F.; Bjork, J.: & Arfors, K.E. (Ch.10): "Pathology of Oxygen," Academic Press, New York, 1982.
3. Hallinel, B. & Gutteridge, M.C.: "Oxygen Toxicity, Oxygen Free Radicals, Transition Metals, and Disease.", J. Biochemistry, 219: 1-14.
4. Hallinel, B,: "Oxygen Radicals: A Common Sense Look at Their Nature & Medical Importance," Medical Biology, 1984, 62: 71-77.
5. French Patent 8605183

Appendix G

Reprinted with permission

Your Cancer Prevention Plan

Reprinted from LIFESPAN-PLUS ©1990 by Rodale Press. Permission granted by Rodale Press, Inc.; Emmaus, PA 18098

Do you know someone with cancer? We'll bet that you do. We'll bet that you do because cancer strikes 3 out of every 4 families in the United States and kills about 500,000 men and women in every year.

Most cancer victims die from cancer of the lung, breast, colon, or prostate. Breast cancer deaths have held steady over the past 30 years, but prostate cancer deaths have increased 9 percent, colon cancer deaths have increased 22 percent in men, and long cancer deaths have increased a shocking 161 percent in men and a horrifying 396 percent in women.

Those increases make cancer the nation's second most common cause of death. But what's causing this epidemic of neoplasmic proliferation?

Most of the time it's things we do to ourselves. We take a 3-inch paper-covered cylinder out of a pack, put one end in our mouths, and set the other end on fire — even when we know that 83 percent of all lung cancer is caused by smoking cigarettes. Or we pull up to a fast-food drive-in, order a bacon double cheeseburger, large fries, and jumbo milkshake — even when we know that the risk of dying from breast cancer increases 40 percent for every extra 1,000 grams of fat we eat a month. Or maybe for breakfast we eat the cute little pink-and-white cereal advertised on Saturday morning cartoons — even when we know that a low-fiber diet is a significant factor in the development of colon cancer.

68 Percent Can Be Prevented

All told, scientists estimate, 35 percent of all cancer deaths are caused by bad diet, 30 percent by smoking, 2 percent by a polluted environment, and 1 percent by food additives.

These numbers add up to the fact that more than 68 percent of all cancer deaths are caused by things we do to ourselves and one another. And that means that every one of these deaths is preventable.

Which ones? In large measure, we can prevent bladder, breast, colon, esophageal, larynx, liver, lung, oral, skin, stomach, and uterine cancer by carefully choosing what we eat, drink, and breathe. The following tips will show us how.

FOODS TO FIGHT CANCER

Eat Bran and Other Fibers

A decade of studies has clearly demonstrated that people who eat a high-fiber diet have a low incidence of cancer — especially colon cancer.

Why? "Fiber appears to dilute intestinal contents and reduces the amount of time carcinogens might spend in your intestines," says the American Cancer Society.

Most people, though, don't eat nearly enough fiber. Current recommendations call for eating 20-30 grams a day, while most of us only get about half that.

If you're looking to increase your fiber intake, try eating foods like whole-grain breads, rice, wheat and bran cereals, popcorn, raisins, peaches, apricots, apples with skin, oranges, strawberries, cherries, potatoes, spinach, peas, tomatoes, kidney beans, carrots, and broccoli.

Eat Less Fat

"Numerous studies have shown that high-fat diets increase the incidence of breast, prostate, and colon cancer," says the American Cancer Society.

So cut down on your total fat intake and really declare war on the saturated fats — the kind of fat that stays solid at room temperature. Most doctors now agree that the amount of fat you consume should equal no more than 30 percent of your total calories.

Start by eating lean meats, skinned poultry, and low-fat dairy products, and bake or broil rather than fry fish, meat, and poultry.

Reach for Vitamin A

Researchers around the world are singing the praises of vitamin A.

- In Canada and India, vitamin A supplements reversed more than half of the oral ulcers that usually lead to oral cancer.
- At the University of Wales College of Medicine, a vitamin A derivative reduced the number of precancerous and cancerous skin growths in 15 patients.
- In China, vaginal suppositories containing

another vitamin A derivative reversed precancerous cervical changes in 26 out of 27 women.

- At the University of Colorado Health Sciences Center, researchers found that retinoic acid, a synthetic form of vitamin A, reduced the growth of cancer cells in a laboratory culture.

Those are only a few of the many positive studies that have surfaced. But a word of caution: High doses of vitamin A can be toxic, so it's not recommended that you take supplements to get this cancer-fighting potential. Instead, eat foods rich in vitamin A.

Look for dark green or deep yellow vegetables such as spinach, tomatoes, or carrots, or fruits such as cantaloupes, apricots, and peaches.

Eat a Carrot a Day

Beta-carotene is the natural pigment found in fruits and vegetables that your body turns into vitamin A. And like vitamin A, it's also been found to help prevent lung cancer.

Researchers at the State University of New York at Buffalo compared the diets of 450 people with lung cancer to the diets of over 900 healthy people. They found that the people with lung cancer had a significantly lower carotene intake than the people without lung cancer. And men with the lowest carotene intake had an 80 percent greater risk than those with the highest intake.

How much carotene would you need to have in your diet to reduce your risk of cancer? Not much. The researchers found the differences in carotene levels was about 6,750 international units — or about the amount of carotene found in one carrot.

Smokers Need Their B's

Since studies show that smokers have lower levels of vitamin B12 and folate than nonsmokers, scientists are beginning to suspect that tobacco smoke may deplete these two essential B vitamins from the cells lining the lung.

Researchers at the University of Alabama at Birmingham decided to clear the air and find out just how these nutrients may play a role in preventing cancer. They studied 73 longtime smokers, all with precancerous cell changes in lung secretions. Half of these smokers received supplements of folate and B12; the other half were given placebos (inactive substances).

After four months, the researchers rechecked the smokers' lung fluids. The fluids of those who took vitamins were found to have less severe precancerous changes than the fluids of those who did not.

You can get B12 by eating lean beef and other meats and certain fish, such as salmon and oysters. Good sources of folate include kidney beans, soybeans, cowpeas, spinach, brewer's yeast, broccoli, and sweet potatoes.

Hold the Bacon

Nitrates have been traditionally used as a way of preserving meat because they act as a preventive against botulism. Trouble is, although they may stop you from getting food poisoning, they may contribute to giving you cancer.

According to the American Cancer Society, in parts of the world where nitrates are common in food and water — Colombia, for instance — stomach and esophageal cancers are common.

In addition, there is chemical evidence that nitrates can enhance nitrosamine formation both in foods and our digestive tract. And nitrosamines have been proven to be potent cancer-causing agents in animals.

Nitrates are found in many processed meat products such as hot dogs, bacon, bologna, and ham. It's best to use these foods in moderation — or skip them altogether.

Or Make It in the Microwave

Researchers have found that microwaving bacon produces fewer cancer-causing nitrosamines than does frying.

How do they know? They cooked up a bunch of bacon. Forty-five seconds of microwaving — the usual amount of time it takes to thoroughly cook a single strip of bacon — produced no nitrosamines. The same amount of time spent in the frying pan produced a significant amount.

Microwaving doesn't make the bacon less fatty, though, even when it's cooked on paper towels. But if you want to reduce your fat as well as your nitrosamines, choose one of the lower-fat bacon substitutes on the marker.

Eat Your Bacon with an Orange Juice Chaser

People who eat vitamin C-rich fruits daily have a lower incidence of cancers of the stomach, esophagus, mouth, larynx, and cervix. There is evidence that it may help prevent colon and lung cancers as well.

The reason vitamin C is so potent against stomach-related cancers apparently is due to its ability to halt the formation of cancer-causing nitrosamines that form in the stomach after eating foods containing nitrates.

Scientists involved in these studies recommend that to get this protective effect you should eat citrus fruits, not take a vitamin C supplement.

That's because they found that the nations and groups of people with the lowest incidence of these cancers get their vitamin C by eating lots of fresh citrus fruits. The possibility exists, they speculate, that there could actually be something in citrus fruit other than just vitamin C that's providing cancer protection.

Calcium Helps Block Colon Cancer

When researchers at the University of Utah School of Medicine compared 231 people with colon cancer against 391 healthy people, they discovered that the people who were cancer-free ate a diet richer in calcium than those with the disease.

The theory behind the study suggests that calcium may slow colon cancer development by binding with the fats and bile acids that could cause bowel tumors.

Open Wide for Vitamin E

Imaging trying to get a hamster to say "Ahhhh." Researchers trying to detect oral cancer at Harvard's School of Dental Medicine spent 28 weeks looking into the gaping jaws of hamsters, trying to detect oral cancer.

What they were doing was treating the hamsters' mouths with a carcinogen combined with a twice-weekly dose of vitamin E. The results after all those weeks? "No evidence whatsoever" of any tumors were found in the hamsters who were given vitamin E. Hamsters given the carcinogen without the vitamin E, though, did show tumor development.

"If vitamin E worked on mouth cancer," says Gerald Shklar, M.D., one of the researchers involved, "you have something that may prevent other cancers as well."

Finnish researchers apparently agree. A ten-year Finnish study that included more than 21,000 men found that those with the highest level of vitamin E had a 36 percent lower risk of cancer than those with the lowest levels of vitamin E.

The reason, they suggest, is that vitamin E is an anti-oxidant, and slower oxidation of body cells may protect against cancer.

"There is good evidence to show that vitamin E can help prevent cancer," concludes Denham Harman, M.D., Ph.D., a vitamin E researcher at the University of Nebraska College of Medicine.

Vitamin E has also been shown to enhance the effectiveness of anticancer drugs used in chemotherapy in rats.

Foods high in vitamin E are wheat germ oil, sunflower seeds and oil, almonds, peanuts, lobster, salmon, soybean oil, and pecans.

Go Easy on the Iron

Researchers at the National Cancer Institute in Washington, D.C., have found that people with high stores of the mineral iron in their body are at greater risk of developing cancer.

Do not take extra iron unless you need to, says Elisabeth Applegate, Ph.D., nutrition director of the University of California at Davis Adult Fitness and Cardiac Rehabilitation Program. If you do feel the need for some "insurance," she suggests you take a multivitamin/mineral supplement, which typically contains the U.S. Recommended Daily Allowance of iron — 18 milligrams.

Most people can get all the iron they need by eating foods rich in the substance, however. Good sources for iron are foods like lean red meat, dark meat poultry, fish, dried beans, whole grains, dried fruit, enriched grain products, and leafy vegetables.

One last tip: Eat foods rich in vitamin C along with meals. It will improve your iron absorption.

Selenium Shows Some Promise

Preliminary studies are showing that too little selenium may increase your chances of getting cancer. In Finland, researchers found that when 143 men with lung cancer where compared to 264 healthy men, those with the least amount of selenium in their blood were also those who had a higher risk of cancer.

At the University of Bonn in West Germany, scientists wanted to find out if selenium would protect people from the most deadly form of skin cancer, malignant melanoma.

When 101 melanoma victims were compared to 57 cancer-free people, the skin cancer sufferers had lower levels of selenium. People with advanced cancer had the least selenium of all.

None of this means you should go out and buy selenium supplements. Because of the possibility of selenium poisoning, the American Cancer Society advises that "the medically unsupervised use of selenium as a food supplement cannot be recommended."

Instead, get your selenium from foods like seafood (especially tuna fish), kidney, liver, grains, nuts, and rice.

Head for the Cabbage Patch

Researchers have been intrigued for years over the possibility that cruciferous vegetables (such as cabbage, brussels sprouts, and broccoli) contain a substance that helps prevent cancer.

At the University of Nebraska Medical Center, for instance, cancer researchers divided a bunch of mice into two groups. One group was given a regular diet, the others were fed diets rich in cabbage or collard greens. At the end of six weeks the mice were injected with breast cancer cells. The result? The mice fed lots of cabbage and greens diet developed fewer tumors.

The evidence is intriguing enough that the American Cancer Society suggests you include cruciferous vegetables in your cancer-prevention diet.

Go Heavy on the Onions, Please

In China, researchers say they've found a link between low cancer rates and foods from the allium family of plants, including onions and garlic.

The Chinese compared a group of 564 stomach cancer patients to a group of 1,131 healthy people. What they found was that the people who reported eating the greatest number of allium vegetables had the fewest cases of stomach cancer.

In fact, people who ate these vegetables the most had only 40 percent as great a risk for stomach cancer as did people who rarely ate them.

And in another study — this one at the Department of Oral Medicine and Oral Pathology in Harvard School of Dental Medicine — onion extract placed in a test tube with cancer cells stopped cancer growth in its tracks., "Tumor growth inhibition began after 24 hours," report the scientists, "and after four days and ten days of incubation, there was a noted decrease in tumor proliferation."

Start a Strawberry Patch

Scientists have found that strawberries contain an acid that can kill cancer-causing compounds. Ellagic acid has been shown to destroy hydrocarbons, one of the chemicals found in tobacco smoke that's known to cause lung cancer.

You'll also find ellagic acid in grapes and Brazil nuts.

Fish Eaters Have Less Cancer

Scientists looking at the diets of people in 32 countries have found that those who eat fish have less cancer.

In countries where breast cancer rates are high, fish consumption is low. On the other hand, in countries like Japan where fish consumption is high, breast cancer rates tend to be low.

The study was conducted by researchers at the Lugdwig Institute for Cancer Research in Toronto, Canada. Scientists there suspect the link between fish and cancer may come about because fish contains omega-3 fatty acids, which have been shown to suppress cancer cells in laboratory tests.

While the results are only preliminary, the school of thought is it wouldn't hurt to try to increase the amount of fish in your diet.

Tea for You

At the National Cancer Center Research Institute in Tokyo, scientists believe that drinking green tea (so named because it's made from green leaves and is unfermented) can inhibit the growth of cancer tumors.

Areas of Japan where green tea is popular have very low cancer death rates. The researchers believe that a compound in the tea — called EGCG — can block tumor-promoting agents.

Rats (not known to actually drink tea) who had EGCG found in the green tea applied to their skin had significantly lower cancer rates than those not treated.

Oriental green tea can be found in stores that sell a wide variety of herbal teas.

Watch Where You're Woking

Stir-fry vegetables may be good for you — but apparently only if you're not doing the frying.

The smoky fumes from high-temperature cooking oils could cause lung cancer, according to a study of Chinese women who use oils in wok cooking.

Wok-using Chinese women have the same lung cancer rate as American women, but they smoke tobacco only half as much, leading researchers to suspect the wok as the woeful cause.

If you cook with a wok, try to keep the oil temperatures down and further protect yourself by woking in a well-ventilated area.

Practice Safe Grilling

Ah! The smell of sizzling burgers can bring out the carnivore in the best of us. Unfortunately, both the smoke and the char create possible cancer-causing compounds that can be deposited on food. Here are some ways to minimize your barbecue risks.

- Pick low-fat meats for the grill. Fat dripping on hot coals creates harmful smoke and flare-ups that can blacken the meat.
- Cover the grill with foil to protect the meat from the smoke and flames. Punch holes in the foil to let the fat drip out.
- Wrap vegetables and fish in foil to preserve their flavors while at the same time protecting them from the smoke.
- Basting foods while they're cooking will help keep them moist. But don't baste with fat, which can cause flare-ups. Instead use lemon juice, wine, or barbeque sauce.
- Poach or microwave poultry or thick meat until partially cooked, then finish it on the grill. This cuts cooking time and reduces exposure to smoke.
- Trim charred parts before eating.

Order Your Ham Fresh

Conventionally smoked foods like hams and some varieties of sausage and fish absorb at least a portion of the tars that rise from incomplete combustion (smoke), according to the American Cancer Society. These tars contain "numerous carcinogens that are similar chemically to the carcinogenic tars in tobacco smoke."

The risk applies primarily to conventionally smoked meats and fish but probably doesn't apply to "liquid smoke" flavoring. If you eat smoked products, the best advice is to do so in moderation.

Eat a Safer Hot Dog

If it's just not the Fourth of July without those weenies cooking on the grill, try to buy hot dogs containing ingredients ascorbic acid, sodium ascorbate, or sodium erythorbate, suggests the American Cancer Society.

Those three ingredients are vitamin C compounds, and they have been added to the food to protect against cancer-causing substances. Look for them in luncheon meats, too.

A CANCER-FREE LIFESTYLE

Root for a Smokeless Society

Here's one irrefutable fact that should come as no surprise: Smoking causes cancer.

In fact, "cigarette smoking is the most important known *preventable* cause of cancer," notes Ronald Ross, M.D., a professor in the Department of Preventive Medicine at the University of Southern California School of Medicine and an associate director of the Kenneth Norris/USC Comprehensive Cancer Center.

And it's never too late to stop — no matter how long you've been smoking. "A person who begins smoking a pack of cigarettes a day at age 20 and stops smoking at age 60 will, by age 70, have one-half the lung cancer risk of the individual who continues to smoke until age 70," says Dr. Ross.

Make the next cigarette you put out your last.

Do It for Her

If none of the other reasons to stop smoking has worked on you, try this one: Wives of smokers are more likely do develop breast cancer than wives of nonsmokers.

An Oregon researcher analyzed information from 50 countries and found that where male death rates from lung cancer are high, female death rates from breast cancer are high, too.

In countries where few men die from lung cancer, breast cancer is also rare. Experts are wondering whether a passive smoking link could explain why breast cancer rates are rising in so many countries.

Too Fat Is Too Risky

Being overweight can increase your chances of developing certain types of cancer.

In a massive 12-year study conducted by the American Cancer Society, researchers found a marked increase in cancers of the uterus, gallbladder, kidney, stomach, colon, and breast associated with obesity.

"When data for men and women 40 percent or more over ideal weight were reviewed, the women were found to have a 55 percent greater risk and the men a 33 percent greater risk of cancer than those of normal body weight," reported the study.

Drink in Moderation

Alcohol consumption has been linked to 3 percent of the overall cancer rate, with cancers of the liver, mouth, throat, esophagus, larynx, rectum, colon, and breast being implicated.

In a study of 106,203 men and women in northern California, for example, researchers found that people who drank more than three alcoholic drinks a day had a three times greater risk of developing rectal cancer than those who never drank.

And a Harvard Medical School survey of the eating and drinking habits of 89,000 women found that those who drank one or more drinks a day increased their risk of developing breast cancer by 50 percent.

Most scientists, however, are quick to say that the alcohol/cancer link is not 100 proof. For one thing, many of the people studied drank *and* smoked. Their choice of drink also varied greatly.

Nevertheless, there is enough evidence to indicate that excessive use of alcohol is a bad idea.

The best advice? If you must drink, do it in moderation.

Get Out and Exercise

Those who exercise most are least likely to get cancer, according to the results of several studies.

In a Harvard study of 17,000 alumni, researchers found that the death rate from cancer was highest in those who exercised the least. Moderate exercisers did better than those who were sedentary, but not as well as the most active alumni.

Even ex-jocks get a benefit from their past life. When 5,398 people were questioned in another study, it was found that former college athletes had a lower lifetime occurrence rate of cancer than nonathletes.

The nonathletes had almost twice the risk of breast cancer and two and a half times the risk of reproductive system cancer as did former athletes.

Another study, this one among 5,138 men and 7,407 women ranging in age from 25 to 74, came to the same conclusion: "Inactive people are at increased risk of cancer."

It's not exactly known why exercise may help you avoid cancer. Some scientists think it may be because exercise reduces obesity. Others think, at least in some women, it may have to do with the fact that exercise reduces estrogen levels. Others feel it may be linked to the simple fact that exercisers generally have a healthier lifestyle.

Whatever the reason, start walking, swimming, riding a bicycle — anything that will get you exercising at least 30 minutes three times a week.

Put Your Drive in Park

A 22-year study of more than 3,000 men suggests that Type-A behavior — hard-driving, impatient, sometimes hostile — may increase the risk of death from almost every type of cancer.

Conducted by David Ragland, Ph.D., a researcher at the School of Public Health at the University of California at Berkeley, and his colleagues, the study found that the Type-A male was 50 percent more likely to die from all types of cancer, except lung cancer, than the laid-back Type-B male. Their lung cancer rates were the same.

The researchers say they are not sure why Type-A's are more cancer-prone, but they speculate that it has more to do with lifestyle than with personality.

Smile, You'll Live Longer

Being depressed could increase your risk of dying from cancer. A study of 2,018 employees at the Western Electric Company near Chicago over a 20-year period reveals that depression may exacerbate cancer — although, fortunately, it doesn't seem to cause it.

Does that mean that happiness will help ensure you'll be around longer? There are plenty of people — including scientists — who say yes. At least, it's the right attitude to have.

TESTING SAVES LIVES
Get a Regular Pap Test

A study of 1,500 older women by scientists at the Mount Sinai School of Medicine in New York reveals that most women over the age of 65 don't have regular Pap tests — and that one-quarter of them have never had one at all.

The American Cancer Society suggests that every woman should have the test — once a year until she's had three negative smears, and thereafter on her doctor's advice — no matter what her age. The five year survival rate for uterine cancer — which a Pap test can detect — is over 85 percent when it's caught and treated early.

The test may be particularly important for older women. Other studies have found that women older than 65 have two to three times the incidence of abnormal smears — which may be an early sign of cervical or endometrial cancer — than younger women.

Ask the Right Questions

Even though the Pap test is one of the most important medical tests a woman will ever have, the American College of Obstetricians and Gynecologists reports that test results are in error 20 percent of the time. That means one out of very five Pap tests may be wrong.

Half of the errors stem from your doctor's cell sampling techniques, while laboratory problems account for the other half.

How can you fight incompetence? According to the American Cancer Society, you can ensure the best possible work from both your doctor and the lab by asking the following questions:

* Where is my Pap smear going to be sent?
* Is it a licensed and accredited lab?
* Will the laboratory have the test rechecked if the results are abnormal?
* Does the lab provide a full written report?
* Does the lab report poor samples as "inadequate for evaluation" or simply as "negative?"

Your questions are guaranteed to keep your doctor on his toes. And *his* questions to the lab will keep them on theirs.

Appendix H

Institutions and Researchers Involved in Health, Nutrition, and Anti-Aging Research

American Cancer Society

American Cancer Society (cruciferous vegetables)

American Dietetic Association — Gail Levey, nutrition spokesperson

American Journal of Cardiology

Columbia University Institute of Human Nutrition — Brian Morgan, Ph.D.

Cornell University — Nobel Laureate James Sumner

Duke University Medical Center — James Crapo

Harvard University Medical School — Eugene Braunwald, Gerald Shklar, M.D.

Johns Hopkins University School of Medicine — Myron Weisfeldt

Lawrence Laboratory at Berkeley — Lester Packer, M.D.

Louisiana State University, Biodynamics Institute — William Pryor

Ludwig Institute for Cancer Research, Toronto

Massachusetts Institute of Technology — Dr. Richard Wurtman, M.D.

Meharry Medical College Nutrition Center — Cyril Enwonwu, Ph.D.

National Academy of Sciences

National Cancer Institute

National Cancer Center Research Institute, Tokyo

National Heart, Lung, and Blood Institute

National Institute on Aging — Edward Schneider

National Research Council

Oklahoma Medical Research Foundation — Paul McKay

Royal College of Physicians — Douglas Model, M.D.

Scripps Clinic and Research Foundation — Charles Cochran

Stanford University — Robert Sapolsky, neuroscientist

State University of New York at Buffalo

Swiss Institute for Experimental Cancer Research — Peter Cerutti

Temple University School of Medicine — Dr. Paul Yanick, biochemist

Texas A&M University — Margeurite M.B. KayUniversity of Texas

University of Alabama at Birmingham

University of Bonn, W. Germany

University of British Columbia — Hans Stich, researcher

University of California at Berkeley School of Public Health — David Ragland, Ph.D.

University of California at Berkeley, School of Public Health — Gladys Block

University of California at Berkeley, Membrane Bioenergetics Group — Bruce Ames, Lester Packer, M.D.

University of California at Los Angeles — Roy Walford, gerontologist

University of California at San Diego — Daniel Steinberg

University of Colorado Health Sciences Center

University of Illinois School of Public Health — Jacob Brody, Dean

University of Iowa School of Medicine

University of Iowa School of Medicine — Robert Clark

University of Michigan Medical Center

University of Michigan Medical Center, Ann Arbor — Stephen Weiss

University of Nebraska College of Medicine — Dr. Denham Harman, M.D.

University of Pennsylvania Center for the Study of Aging — Vincent Cristofalo, director

University of Southern Alabama School of Medicine — Joseph McCord, biochemist

University of Southern California School of Medicine — Ronald Ross, M.D.

University of Texas at San Antonio — Edward Masoro, physiologist

University of Utah School of Medicine

University of Wales College of Medicine

University of Washington — George M. Martin, pathologist

University of Wisconsin

University of Wisconsin Biogerontology Laboratory — Everett Smith, Ph.D.

USDA Human Nutrition Research Center on Aging, Tufts University — Jeffrey Blumberg, Ph.D.

USDA Laboratories, Beltsville — Frederick Khachik, scientist

BIBLIOGRAPHY

Abderhalden, R. Clinical Enzymology. New York: Van Nostrand, 1961.

Adams, Rex. Miracle Medicine Foods. New York: Parker Publishing, 1977.

Airola, Ph.D., N.D., Paavo. Are You Confused: The Authoritative Answers to Controversial Questions. Arizona: Health Plus Publishers, 1971.

Airola, Ph.D., N.D., Paavo. There Is A Cure for Arthritis. New York: Parker Publishing, 1968.

Allee Ph.D., John Gage. Webster's New Encyclopedia of Dictionaries. Ottenheimer Publishers, 1986.

Asplund, Åke. Searching the Source of Life and Vitality. Thailand: Sanomin SDN, 1991.

Balch, M.D., James and Phyllis Balch, C.N.C. Prescription for Nutritional Healing. New York: Avery Publishers, 1990.

Beverly, Cal and June Gunden. New Health Tips Encyclopedia. Georgia: FC&A Publishing, 1992.

Bliznakov M.D., Dr. Emile and Gerald L. Hunt. The Miracle Nutrient: Coenzyme Q10. New York: Bantam, 1987.

Bricklin, Mark. The Practical Encyclopedia of Natural Healing. Emmaus, PA: Rodale Press, 1976.

Bricklin, Mark. Prevention Magazine's Complete Nutrition Reference Handbook. Emmaus, PA: Rodale Press, 1992.

Carlotti, Pierre, Denise Gabrielle. "The Cellular Aging Process and Free Radicals." Drug and Cosmetic Industry Journal. France: Sederma, 2/89, p. 22(3).

Carper, Jean. "Free Radical Fighters." Washington,DC: Washington Post, 6/20/89, p. WH20 col. 2.

Clayman, M.D., Charles. Practical Family Health. New York: Reader's Digest Association.

Chabner, Davi-Ellen. The Language of Medicine. Philadelphia: W. B. Saunders Co., 1985.

C.R. Acad. Sc. Paris of 1964. Prevention Magazine. Emmaus, PA: Rodale Press, July 1972.

Davis, Adelle. Let's Get Well. New York: Harcourt, Brace & World, 1965.

DeCava, J. "What Is a Vitamin." Journal of the National Academy of Research Biochemists, vol. 6:11, 1986.

Dessy, R., J. Dillard, L. Taylor. Bio-organic Chemistry, Advanced Chemistry, Series 100. American Chemistry Society, 1971.

De vries, Jan. Body Energy. Edinburgh, England: Mainstream Publishing, 1989.

Diamond, Harvey and Marilyn. Fit For Life. New York: Warner Books, 1987.

"Diet, Nutrition and Cancer." Washington, DC: National Academy Press, 1982, pp. 1-8.

Dunne, Lavon. Nutrition Almanac. New York: McGraw-Hill, 1990.

Dyke, S. F. "The Chemistry of Vitamins." Interscience. New York: John Wiley, 1965.

Editors of Consumer Guide. Complete Book of Vitamins and Minerals. Illinois: Publications International, 1988.

Eichenlaub, M.D., Dr. John. A Minnesota Doctor's Home Remedies for Common and Uncommon Ailments. New Jersey: Prentice Hall, 1960.

Enstrom, J.E., L.E. Kanim, M.A. Klein. "Vitamin C intake and mortality among a sample of the United States population." Epidemiology, 192, 3:194-202.

Fahy, Ph.D., Dr. Gregory. "Life Extension Benefits of Coenzyme Q10". Published research article from archive files.

"Food and Nutrition Research News," Washington, D.C.: U.S. Department of Agriculture, Oct-Dec 1987.

Foote, C.S., R.F. del Maestro, J. Bjork, K.E. Arfors. Pathology of Oxygen. New York: Academic Press, 1982.

Gardner, M.D., Dr. Weston and William Osburn. Anatomy of the Human Body. Philadelphia: W. B. Saunders Co., 1978.1

Hagiwara, Yoshihide. Green Barley Essence. New Canaan, CT: Keats Publishing, 1985.

Hallinel, B. and M.C. Gutteridge. "Oxygen Toxicity, Oxygen Free Radicals, Transition Metals, and Disease." Journal of Biochemistry.

Hallinel, B. "Oxygen Radicals: A Common Sense Look At Their Nature & Medical Importance". Medical Biology. 1984.

Hallowell, Michael. Herbal Healing. Bath, England: Ashgrove Press, 1985.

Hanson, W. Biomolecular Applications, Bio-Energetic Approach to Healing: A Handbook for Physicians. EPP Publications, 1988.

Hanson, W. "Molecular Biology in Preventive Medicine." Journal of the International Academy of Preventive Medicine, vol. 5:12, 1983.

Health News and Review. "Ascorbic Acid: Biological functions and Relation to Cancer." A seminar sponsored by the National Cancer Institute and the National Institute of Digestive and Kidney Diseases, Washington, D.C., 1990. New Canaan, CT: Keats Publishing, July/August 1991.

Hendler, M.D., Ph.D., Sheldon. The Complete Guide to Anti-Aging Nutrients. New York: Simon and Schuster, 1985.

Hoffer, A. Research article in the New England Journal of Medicine. 1971.

Horwitt, Max. "Vitamin E 1986 Research Abstracts." Vitamin E Research and Information Service. LaGrange, IL: Henkel Corporation, 1986.

Howell, Edward. Enzyme Nutrition. Wayne, NJ: Avery Publishing, 1987.

Howell, Dr. Edward. Food Enzymes for Health & Longevity. CT: Omangod Press, 1980.

Hunt, Gerald. "Coenzyme Q10 Miracle Nutrient." Omni Science Magazine.

Israel, Richard. The Natural Pharmacy Product Guide. New York: Avery Publishers, 1991.

Jarvis,RN,C,MSN,FNP, Carolyn. Physical Examination and Health Assessment. Philadelphia: W. B. Saunders.

Jawetz, M.D., Ph.D., Ernest, Joseph Melnick, Ph.D., Edward Adelberg, Ph.D. Jawetz, Melnick & Adelberg's Medical Microbiology. Norwalk, CT: Appleton & Lange.

Jensen, Dr. Bernard. Foods That Heal. New York: Avery Publishing, 1988.

Kamei, M. "The Distribution and Content of Ubiquinone in Foods." International Journal of Nutritional Research. 1986.

Kadans, Ph.D., Joseph. Encyclopedia of Fruits, Vegetables, Nuts and Seeds for Healthful Living. New York: Parker Publishing, 1973.

Kanungo, M.S. Biochemistry of Aging. London: Academic Press, 1980.

Klenner, F. R. Journal of International Academy of Preventive Medicine. 1974.

Klenner, F. R. Journal of Applied Nutrition. 1971.

Kouchakoff, P. "The Influence of Cooking Food on the Blood Formula of Man." Proceedings of the First International Congress of Microbiology, Paris, 1930.

Kumler, Dr. Warren. "Biochemical Individuality and the Case for Supplemental Vitamins." University of California School of Pharmacy. American Pharmaceutical Association, 1979.

Lazarus, Pat. "The Purest Lecithin Yet." Let's Live Magazine, August 1980.

Lee, Dr. William H. Coenzyme Q10, A Good Health Guide. New Canaan, CT: Keats Publishing, 1987.

Lenaz, G. Coenzyme Q10: Biochemistry, Bioenergetics and Clinical Applications. New York: John Wiley, 1985.

Ludington, M.D., Aileen. Bottom Line Personal. New York: Boardroom Reports, 10/15/92.

Lynes, Barry. The Healing of Cancer. Ontario, Canada: Marcus Books, 1989.

Marx, Jean L. "Oxygen Free Radical Linked to Many Diseases." Science, 1/30/87, p. 529(3).

Meier, Larry. "UCLA Study Credits Vitamin C With 6 Year Life Extension" (1992), "Seven Key Energies of Life and Longevity" (1992), "Antioxidant Enzymes" (1989), and "Bio-energetic vs. Synthetic-Chemical Nutrition" (1990) by Dr. Paul Yanick (all used with permission). Federal Way, WA: Life Enthusiast Co-Op, Quantum Advance International, and Creative Insights.

Meyeroff, Wendy. "Winning A-C-E's." Weight Watchers, 4/91, p. 22(2).

Mindell, Earl. Vitamin Bible. New York: Warner Books, 1991.

Morehouse, Dr. Laurence, and Leonard Gross. Total Fitness in 30 Minutes a Week. New York: Pocket Books, 1976.

Murray, Ph.D., Patrick, W. Lawrence Drew, M.D., Ph.D., George Kobayashi, Ph.D., John Thompson, Jr., Ph.D. Medical Microbiology. St. Louis: The C.V. Mosby Company.

Murray, R. "Natural versus Synthetic - Life versus Death - Truth versus the Lie." The Clinical Nutritionist, vol. 2:5, 1982.

New York Public Library. The New York Public Library Desk Reference. New York: Webster's Press, 1989.

Nutrition News, 1987, vol. X, no. 8.

Pearson, Durk and Sandy Shaw. Life Extension. New York: Warner Books, 1982.

Pearson, Durk and Sandy Shaw. Life Extension Companion. New York: Warner Books, 1984.

Prevention Magazine. The Doctor's Book of Home Remedies. Emmaus, PA: Rodale Press, 1990.

Prevention Magazine. Future Youth: How To Reverse the Aging Process. Emmaus, PA: Rodale Press, 1987.

Prevention Magazine. Lifespan Plus: 900 Natural Techniques to Live Longer. Emmaus, PA: Rodale Press, 1990.

Prostabrit press release. "Silent Sufferers — Male Prostate Problems Affect 50% of Men Over 50". Switzerland: Cernitin SA, 1992.

Raloff, J. "Vitamin E Fights Radicals - Again and Again." Science News, 5/27/89, p. 327(1).

Rodale, J.I. The Complete Book of Vitamins. Emmaus, PA: Rodale Press, 1971.

Rodale, J.I. Prevention Method for Better Health. Emmaus, PA: Rodale Press, 1970.

Roitt, MA,DSc, FRCPath, FRS, Ivan and Peter Delves, Ph.D. Encyclopedia of Immunology. New York: Academic Press.

Seibold, M.S., Ronald. Cereal Grass: What's In It for You. Lawrence, Kansas: Wilderness Community Education Foundation, 1990.

Shimer, Porter. "Fountain of Youth." Organic Gardening, 12/88, p. 62(4).

Silberner, J. "Cell Aging: A Process of Oxidation." Science News, 4/19/86, p. 247.

Simone, M.D., Charles. Cancer and Nutrition. New York: Avery Publishers, 1992.

Singleton, Paul and Diana Sainsbury. Dictionary of Microbiology and Molecular Biology. New York: John Wiley & Sons.

Somer M.A., R.D, Elizabeth. "Fighting the Radicals." Shape, 7/92, p. 32(2).

Stedman, Nancy. "Ways To Stay Younger Longer." Reader's Digest, 6/88, p. 21(6).

Stedman, Nancy. "10 Ways To Slow Down Aging." Woman's Day, 1/20/87, p.40(4).

Steiner, R. F. Chemical Foundations of Molecular Biology. New York: Van Nostrand, 1965.

Swope, Dr. Mary Ruth. Green Leaves of Barley. Arizona: Swope Enterprises, 1990.

"The 200 Year Old Man." Longevity Magazine, August 1992.

Todd, M.D., Gary Price. Nutrition, Health, and Disease. Donning Co., 1985.

Vandeman, G. The Miracle of Hunza. Thousand Oaks, 1982.

Van Fleet, James. A Doctor's Proven New Way to Conquer Rheumatism and Arthritis. New Jersey: Prentice Hall, 1992.

Werbach, M.D., Melvyn. Nutritional Influences on Illness. CT: Keats Publishing, 1987.

Wigmore, Ann. Be Your Own Doctor: A Positive Guide to Natural Living. New Jersey: Avery Publishing, 1982.

Wigmore, Ann. Recipes for Longer Life. New Jersey: Avery Publishing, 1978.

Wodehouse, Ph.D., R.P. Pollen Grains: Their Structure, Identification and Significance in Science and Medicine. New York: Hafner Publishing, 1959.

Yanick, Ph.D., Paul. Guidelines to Better Health: A Bioenergetic Approach. Pennsylvania: EPP Publications, 1988.

Yanick, Ph.D., Paul. Manual of Neurohormonal Regulation. New York: Biological Energetics Press, 1992.